Immigrant Health

Editors

FERN R. HAUCK
CARINA M. BROWN

PRIMARY CARE:
CLINICS IN OFFICE PRACTICE

www.primarycare.theclinics.com

Consulting Editor
JOEL J. HEIDELBAUGH

March 2021 • Volume 48 • Number 1

ELSEVIER

1600 John F. Kennedy Boulevard • Suite 1800 • Philadelphia, Pennsylvania, 19103-2899

http://www.theclinics.com

PRIMARY CARE: CLINICS IN OFFICE PRACTICE Volume 48, Number 1
March 2021 ISSN 0095-4543, ISBN-13: 978-0-323-79251-6

Editor: Katerina Heidhausen
Developmental Editor: Laura Fisher

Primary Care: Clinics in Office Practice (ISSN: 0095-4543) is published quarterly by Elsevier Inc., 360 Park Avenue South, New York, NY 10010-1710. Months of issue are March, June, September, and December. Periodicals postage paid at New York, NY and additional mailing offices. Subscription prices are $261.00 per year (US individuals), $649.00 (US institutions), $100.00 (US students), $303.00 (Canadian individuals), $688.00 (Canadian institutions), $100.00 (Canadian students), $357.00 (international individuals), $688.00 (international institutions), and $175.00 (international students). Foreign air speed delivery is included in all *Clinics* subscription prices. All prices are subject to change without notice. POSTMASTER: Send address changes to *Primary Care: Clinics in Office Practice*, Elsevier Periodicals Customer Service, 11830 Westline Industrial Drive, St. Louis, MO 63146. Customer Service Health Sciences Division, Subscription Customer Service, 3251 Riverport Lane, Maryland Heights, MO 63043. **Customer Service: 1-800-654-2452 (U.S. and Canada); 314-447-8871 (outside U.S. and Canada). Fax: 314-447-8029. E-mail: journalscustomerservice-usa@elsevier.com (for print support); journalsonlinesupport-usa@elsevier.com (for online support).**

Reprints. For copies of 100 or more, of articles in this publication, please contact the Commercial Reprints Department, Elsevier Inc., 360 Park Avenue South, New York, NY 10010-1710. Tel. 212-633-3874; Fax: 212-633-3820; E-mail: reprints@elsevier.com.

Primary Care: Clinics in Office Practice is covered in *MEDLINE/PubMed (Index Medicus)* and *EMBASE/Excerpta Medica, Current Contents/Clinical Medicine,* and *ISI/BIOMED.*

Contributors

CONSULTING EDITOR

JOEL J. HEIDELBAUGH, MD, FAAFP, FACG
Clinical Professor, Departments of Family Medicine and Urology, Director of Medical Student Education and Clerkship Director, Department of Family Medicine, University of Michigan Medical School, Ann Arbor, Michigan, USA; Ypsilanti Health Center, Ypsilanti, Michigan, USA

EDITORS

FERN R. HAUCK, MD, MS, FAAFP
Spencer P. Bass, MD Twenty-First Century Professor of Family Medicine, Professor of Public Health Sciences, Director of Research and Faculty Development, Director, International Family Medicine Clinic, Department of Family Medicine, University of Virginia Health System, Charlottesville, Virginia, USA

CARINA M. BROWN, MD
Assistant Professor, Department of Family Medicine, Cone Health Family Medicine Residency, The University of North Carolina at Chapel Hill, Greensboro, North Carolina, USA

AUTHORS

NICOLE CHOW AHRENHOLZ, MD
Attending Physician and Clinic Education Director, International Medicine Clinic, Harborview Medicine Center, Clinical Assistant Professor of Medicine, University of Washington School of Medicine, Seattle, Washington, USA

CLAUDIA W. ALLEN, PhD, JD, ABPP
Director of Behavioral Science, Professor, Department of Family Medicine, University of Virginia, Charlottesville, Virginia, USA

SCOTT BLAND, DO
Chief Resident, Cone Health Family Medicine Residency, Greensboro, North Carolina, USA

MICAH BRICKHILL-ATKINSON
Medical Student, Department of Family Medicine, University of Virginia School of Medicine, Charlottesville, Virginia, USA

AMY C. BROWN, MD, MHS
Associate Professor, Department of Pediatrics, University of Virginia, Charlottesville, Virginia, USA

CARINA M. BROWN, MD
Assistant Professor, Department of Family Medicine, Cone Health Family Medicine Residency, The University of North Carolina at Chapel Hill, Greensboro, North Carolina, USA

ELIZABETH CARPENTER, RN, BSN
RN Care Coordinator, International Family Medicine Clinic, Department of Family Medicine, University of Virginia, Charlottesville, Virginia, USA

REBEKAH COMPTON, DNP, RN, FNP-C
Director, Quality Improvement, Department of Family Medicine, University of Virginia, Charlottesville, Virginia, USA

SARAH N. DALRYMPLE, MD
Assistant Professor, Department of Family Medicine, University of Virginia, Charlottesville, Virginia, USA

BRITTANY DIVITO, MPH, MSN, FNP-BC
Family Nurse Practitioner, Department of Family Medicine, District Medical Group/Valleywise, Refugee Family/Internal Medicine Clinic, Phoenix, Arizona, USA

CATHERINE E. ELMORE, PhD(c), MSN, RN, CNL
School of Nursing, University of Virginia, Charlottesville, Virginia, USA

VINCENT GIRARD, BHSc
Medical Doctor 2022, University of Ottawa, Ottawa, Ontario, Canada

KIM S. GRISWOLD, MD, MPH, FAAFP
Professor of Family Medicine, Psychiatry and Public Health and the Health Professions, Department of Family Medicine, Jacobs School of Medicine and Biomedical Sciences, Buffalo, New York, USA

FERN R. HAUCK, MD, MS, FAAFP
Spencer P. Bass, MD Twenty-First Century Professor of Family Medicine, Professor of Public Health Sciences, Director of Research and Faculty Development, Director, International Family Medicine Clinic, Department of Family Medicine, University of Virginia Health System, Charlottesville, Virginia, USA

ALISON N. HUFFSTETLER, MD
Assistant Professor, Department of Family Medicine and Population Health, Virginia Commonwealth University, Richmond, Virginia, USA

KRISTINA JOHNSON, MD
Assistant Professor, Department of Family Medicine, University of Virginia, Charlottesville, Virginia, USA

SARAH KIMBALL, MD
Co-Director, Immigrant and Refugee Health Center, Boston Medical Center, Assistant Professor of Medicine, Boston University School of Medicine, Boston, Massachusetts, USA

DIANNE M. LOOMIS, DNP, FNP-BC
Associate Clinical Professor, Emeritus, University at Buffalo, School of Nursing, Buffalo, New York, USA

MEGAN H. MENDEZ MILLER, DO
Assistant Professor, Department of Family and Community Medicine, Penn State Health, Milton S. Hershey Medical Center, Hershey, Pennsylvania, USA

BRIANNA MOYER, MD
Associate Director, Family and Community Medicine Residency Program, Penn Medicine Lancaster General Health, Lancaster, Pennsylvania, USA

PATRICIA A. PASTORE, MSN, FNP-BC
Retired, Grand Island, New York, USA

COLLEEN PAYTON, PhD, MPH
Assistant Professor of Public Health, School of Nursing and Public Health, Moravian College, Bethlehem, Pennsylvania, USA

KEVIN POTTIE, MD, CCFP, MCISc, FCFP
Professor, Department of Family Medicine, School of Epidemiology Public Health and Preventive Medicine, University of Ottawa, Ottawa, Ontario, Canada

SARAH I. RAMIREZ, MD
Assistant Professor, Department of Family and Community Medicine, Penn State Health, Milton S. Hershey Medical Center, Hershey, Pennsylvania, USA

KELLY REESE, MD
Associate Director, Family and Community Medicine Residency Program, Penn Medicine Lancaster General Health, Lancaster, Pennsylvania, USA

NADIA SAIF, MD, MPH
Resident Physician, University of Virginia Family Medicine Residency, Charlottesville, Virginia, USA

SARAH SEIFU, MD, MS
Resident Physician, University of Virginia Department of Family Medicine, Charlottesville, Virginia, USA

SHRUTI SIMHA, MD, MPH
Tim and Carolynn Rice Center for Child and Adolescent Health, Cone Health, Greensboro, USA; Adjunct Faculty, Department of Pediatrics, The University of North Carolina at Chapel Hill, Chapel Hill, North Carolina, USA

RACHEL TALAVLIKAR, MD
Clinical Lecturer, Department of Family Medicine, Cumming School of Medicine, University of Calgary, Family Physician, Mosaic Refugee Health Clinic, Calgary, Alberta, Canada

JOSEPH S. TAN, PhD
Assistant Professor, Department of Family Medicine, University of Virginia, Charlottesville, Virginia, USA

ERICA UHLMANN, MPH
Medical Case Manager, International Rescue Committee, Charlottesville, Virginia, USA

JEFFREY WALDEN, MD
Associate Professor of Family Medicine, College of Health Sciences, University of Montana, Missoula, Montana, USA

TAYLOR WALTERS, MPH
Health Liaison, International Rescue Committee, Richmond, Virginia, USA

MARK L. WIELAND, MD, MPH
Associate Professor of Medicine, Community Internal Medicine, Mayo Clinic, Rochester, Minnesota, USA

Contents

Foreword: The Time is NOW   xiii

Joel J. Heidelbaugh

Preface: Caring for Refugees and Immigrants: Challenges and Opportunities   xv

Fern R. Hauck and Carina M. Brown

Caring for the Forcibly Displaced   1

Jeffrey Walden

> Immigration, and health issues surrounding the immigration status of pa-
> tients, remains much in the media forefront and will likely remain so in
> the future due to ongoing political challenges. Although precise definitions
> of immigrants, refugees, and asylum seekers remain vitally important when
> framing discussions around immigration, all newcomers face health chal-
> lenges. By educating themselves about these issues, health care profes-
> sionals can better care for their patients, no matter their specialty.

Refugee Medical Screening   9

Kelly Reese and Brianna Moyer

> The domestic medical examination of newly arrived refugees is a
> comprehensive medical visit. It includes a review of the overseas med-
> ical examination and a thorough medical and immigration history. It
> should include laboratory testing for infectious diseases, pregnancy,
> and other conditions as recommended by the Centers for Disease Con-
> trol and Prevention and resettlement state, as well as a comprehensive
> physical examination with attention paid to conditions known to specific
> refugee groups. It should also include vaccinations for age-appropriate
> vaccine-preventable diseases. The concept of preventive care should
> be introduced, and future visits should be scheduled for preventive
> care.

Effective Communication with Refugees and Immigrants   23

Carina M. Brown, Scott Bland, and Nadia Saif

> Immigrant and refugee patients may have limited English proficiency.
> Effective use of professional interpreter services reduces clinically sig-
> nificant errors and increases the quality of care. A multitude of profes-
> sional interpreter services are available, and clinicians should carefully
> select the preferred modality of interpretation based on the type of
> encounter. Ad hoc interpreters, such as family members, are least
> preferred because of concerns of privacy and evidence of poorer out-
> comes. Children less than 18 years of age should only be used as inter-
> preters in emergency situations. Professional telephonic, video, or in-
> person interpreters each have distinct advantages in specific clinical
> situations.

Cultural Considerations in Caring for Refugees and Immigrants   35

Joseph S. Tan and Claudia W. Allen

> This article describes the different ways culture affects health care, in terms of patient-related factors, health care provider–related factors, and health care system–related factors. This article also reviews interventions and best practices that draw on the incorporation of culture into health care and that thus may be effective for building cross-cultural understanding between providers and their immigrant and refugee patients.

Common Infectious Diseases   45

Kevin Pottie and Vincent Girard

> The initial assessment of immigrant and refugee patients, including which health concerns to address and which infectious diseases may benefit from early screening, may present challenges to clinicians. Evidence-based research suggests certain infectious diseases should be screened for and treated in refugees. Overseas refugee preemptive treatment programs have reduced the burden of some diseases but have not removed the value of in-country screening programs. This article provides discussion of a series of common tropical and infectious diseases providing refugee and geographic contexts and links to international resources that have been developed to improve the care of newly arriving immigrants and refugees.

Impact of COVID-19 on Resettled Refugees   57

Micah Brickhill-Atkinson and Fern R. Hauck

> Refugees are among the world's most vulnerable people, and COVID-19 presents novel threats to their well-being. Suspension of resettlement prolongs persecution for those accepted but not yet relocated to a host country and delays family reunification. For new arrivals, pandemic-related modifications to resettlement services impair smooth transitions. Refugees are additionally more vulnerable to economic hardship, COVID-19 infection, and mental illness exacerbations. Communication barriers make telehealth access uniquely difficult, and children lose the school environment that is essential for their adaptation in a new country. Providers can mitigate pandemic-related harms by assessing barriers, disseminating information, and advocating for inclusive policies.

Common Hematologic, Nutritional, Asthma/Allergic Conditions and Lead Screening/ Management   67

Brittany DiVito, Rachel Talavlikar, and Sarah Seifu

> This article describes hematologic, nutritional, allergic/asthmatic conditions, lead screening, and management of these among immigrants and refugees. Some of these conditions present more frequently or differently in the newcomer population. Early identification and treatment are key to improving health outcomes. Screening and treatment suggested in this article are based on current guidelines and are intended for primary care providers who are caring for refugee and immigrant patients, especially within a medical home. Special considerations include level of education, instruction, demonstration, and cultural humility.

Preventive Care and Management of Chronic Diseases in Immigrant Adults   83

Colleen Payton, Sarah Kimball, Nicole Chow Ahrenholz, and Mark L. Wieland

> Immigrants may have variable access to chronic disease screening and treatment in their countries of origin and host country, often limited by their immigration status. Immigrants face barriers to chronic disease management and preventive care, including health insurance access, linguistic challenges, lack of culturally sensitive care, limited records, and acculturation. Health care providers should prioritize chronic disease screening and follow up regularly to encourage preventive care and self-management of chronic disease.

Preventive Care in Children and Adolescents   99

Shruti Simha and Amy C. Brown

> This article describes the current state of migration of immigrant children into the United Sates and the various categories of immigrant children, including refugees, asylum seekers, unaccompanied minors, adoptees, and Special Immigrant Visa holders, hereafter called immigrant children. It focuses on guidelines for medical screening and management of newcomer immigrant children and adolescents and their ongoing preventive care. This article also addresses challenges unique to immigrant children and adolescents and the importance of culturally sensitive anticipatory guidance.

Women's Health and Gender-Specific Considerations   117

Alison N. Huffstetler, Sarah I. Ramirez, Sarah N. Dalrymple, and Megan H. Mendez Miller

> Women's health is largely influenced by cultural beliefs, local traditions, and access to care across the world. Immigrant and refugee women experience health in varied ways; prior experiences with health care and beliefs about health should be explored with women on their arrival to the United States. Topics that should be discussed include menstrual practices, contraception and beliefs about family planning, prior screening for preventable diseases, pregnancies and experiences with childbirth, sexual assault and trauma, and history of traditional practices, including female genital mutilation (dependent on area of origin).

Mental Health and Illness   131

Kim S. Griswold, Dianne M. Loomis, and Patricia A. Pastore

> Circumstances forcing individuals and families to flee set the stage for disruptions in mental health and forge resilience. Individual characteristics and conditions premigration, perimigration, and postmigration influence health, mental health, care-seeking behavior, and stages of well-being and successful resettlement. Primary care providers have strategies to promote mental well-being, including focusing on resilience and social determinants of health. Integrated or collaborative care models are ideal for delivering optimum care for refugee and immigrant communities. Connecting primary and behavioral care promotes a team approach; provides comprehensive, whole-person care; and relies on participation of patients and families.

Special Issues in Immigrant Medicine 147

Kristina Johnson, Elizabeth Carpenter, and Taylor Walters

Immigrants enrich the United States through economic contributions and unique perspectives. Immigrants find themselves navigating a new culture, a complicated health care system, unfamiliar social programs, and an ever-changing policy environment. They may be discouraged by unmet expectations of life in the United States, changing family dynamics, and discrimination. Screening for the social determinants of health is crucial, as not all patients will proactively seek the advice of their health care provider for these issues. Health care providers can assist and empower immigrants to navigate these challenges, as well as serve as advocates on a broader scale.

Models of Health Care: Interprofessional Approaches to Serving Immigrant Populations 163

Catherine E. Elmore, Rebekah Compton, and Erica Uhlmann

Developing an integrated model of health care for refugees, asylees, immigrants, and special immigrant visa holders requires a multifaceted approach due to their unique and complex health care needs. This article provides an in-depth understanding of the components necessary to develop a model of care addressing the needs of immigrants and to share opportunities and challenges associated with these models. This includes highlighting population- and individual-level factors important to caring for immigrant populations, providing guidance on creating a model of care that addresses these factors, and describing established clinics that exemplify various models of care.

PRIMARY CARE:
CLINICS IN OFFICE PRACTICE

FORTHCOMING ISSUES

June 2021
LGBTQ+ Health
Jessica Lapinski and Kristine Diaz, *Editors*

September 2021
Common Pediatric Issues in Primary Care
Luz M. Fernandez and Jonathan Becker, *Editors*

December 2021
Office-Based Procedures: Part I
Joseph Lane Wilson, *Editor*

RECENT ISSUES

December 2020
Nephrology
Parvathi Perumareddi, *Editor*

September 2020
Immunizations
Margot Savoy, *Editor*

June 2020
Adolescent Medicine
Benjamin Silverberg, *Editor*

SERIES OF RELATED INTEREST

Medical Clinics (http://www.medical.theclinics.com)

THE CLINICS ARE AVAILABLE ONLINE!
Access your subscription at:
www.theclinics.com

PRIMARY CARE:
CLINICS IN OFFICE PRACTICE
The Clinics.com

FORTHCOMING ISSUES

June 2021
LGBTQ+ Health
Jessica Lapinski and Kristine Diaz, Editors

September 2021
Common Pediatric Issues in Primary Care
Luz M. Fernandez and Jonathan Becker (editor)

December 2021
Office based Procedures: Part 1
Joseph Lane Wilson, Editor

RECENT ISSUES

December 2020
Health...ology
Parviz Feroze-Ahn, Editor

September 2020
Immunizations
Margot Savoy, Editor

June 2020
Adolescent Medicine
Benjamin Silverberg, Editor

SERIES OF RELATED INTEREST

Medical Clinics http://www.medical.theclinics.com

Foreword
The Time is NOW

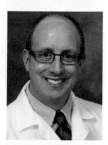

Joel J. Heidelbaugh, MD, FAAFP, FACG
Consulting Editor

As I write this foreword, the 2020 Presidential Election is only 3 short weeks away, and we are in the throes of the COVID-19 global pandemic. Similar to previous elections, health care provisions for Americans will be a top consideration for all voters. In the last decade, the United States has seen a dramatic influx of immigrants and refugees from around the world, as well as the inherent challenges in providing adequate health care for them. These challenges come with many barriers in policy, poor understanding of inherent cultural beliefs, and often insufficient training for health care providers across all disciplines of medicine.

A few months ago, I read an interesting and very well-written article in *The Lancet* entitled, "Challenges for immigrant health in the USA—the road to crisis."[1] It absolutely blew me away. The article provides a very detailed account of US policies past and present that put immigrant health and health care at risk, as well as the many barriers that we face in providing successful health care for this population. While we commonly focus on the challenges of providing health care to the patients we see in our clinics, we often don't consider the missed opportunities for health care for the patients whom we <u>don't</u> see. In some cases, these individuals are the ones with greatest need, and often greatest fear of risk of deportation. This is an exciting time for health care providers to play an influential role in shaping health care law and public policy on both the state and the federal levels.

I would like to sincerely thank Dr Fern R. Hauck and Dr Carina M. Brown for their outstanding work in creating a very timely and important issue of articles dedicated to immigrant and refugee health. I cannot understate the importance of this body of work, as well as the vast amount of knowledge I have gained from reading the articles herein. I would also like to acknowledge the many talented authors who contributed to this issue of *Primary Care: Clinics in Office Practice*. To date, no comparative reference of this magnitude and quality exists. It is our hope that while this issue augments the knowledge and skill of our health care providers as well as the quality of health care

Prim Care Clin Office Pract 48 (2021) xiii–xiv
https://doi.org/10.1016/j.pop.2020.12.002
0095-4543/21/© 2020 Published by Elsevier Inc.

primarycare.theclinics.com

for our immigrants and refugees, that it serves as a blueprint that can spawn advocacy, innovation, research, and policy. The time is NOW to change the future.

Joel J. Heidelbaugh, MD, FAAFP, FACG
Departments of Family Medicine and Urology
University of Michigan Medical School
Ann Arbor, MI, USA

Ypsilanti Health Center
200 Arnet Suite 200
Ypsilanti, MI 48198, USA

E-mail address:
jheidel@umich.edu

REFERENCE

1. Khullar D, Chokshi DA. Challenges for immigrant health in the USA—the road to crisis. Lancet 2019;393:2168–74.

Preface

Caring for Refugees and Immigrants: Challenges and Opportunities

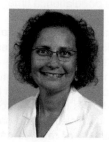 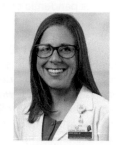

Fern R. Hauck, MD, MS, FAAFP   Carina M. Brown, MD

Editors

Refugees, immigrants, and asylum seekers are moving throughout the world in record numbers, bringing innovation, cultural enhancement, and diversity to their destinations. Refugees and asylum seekers flee their country of origin in hopes of a better, safer life in the country of resettlement. Immigrants travel to a new country for a variety of reasons, many reuniting with family or seeking employment or education. These diverse individuals contribute to society in meaningful ways through the arts, culture, science, and multiple other facets of life, as well as working arduous and lower-paid positions seen as less desirable by many. As primary care clinicians, we have the opportunity to provide comprehensive medical care to individuals at risk for poor health outcomes. The experience of health care abroad is varied, typically one of intermittent, acute care without reliable access to high-quality primary care to prevent and treat chronic medical conditions.

Caring for newly arrived individuals presents a challenge for primary care providers, but also an opportunity to improve the health and well-being of those disproportionately affected by poor health outcomes. Primary care for refugee, immigrant, and asylee (asylees are individuals who have been granted asylum) families involves a multidisciplinary and multiagency approach with numerous stakeholders. Primary care clinicians can provide leadership and guidance to ensure high-quality, timely care and serve as the first contact for the health care system. Working with this team of community agencies, public health officials, social workers, and consultants allows for holistic, comprehensive care of the entire family.

Within this issue, you will find a wide breadth of topics focused on the primary care of refugees, immigrants, and asylees. Walden provides an overview of migration from a global perspective with a moving story of one family's journey and the challenges

Prim Care Clin Office Pract 48 (2021) xv–xvi
https://doi.org/10.1016/j.pop.2020.12.001
0095-4543/21/© 2020 Published by Elsevier Inc.

and rewards of providing health care to refugees. Reese and Moyer comprehensively discuss the domestic screening examination and subsequent preventive health measures required to attain citizenship for refugees. Brown and coauthors highlight the importance of interpretation and translation services, followed by a discussion of cultural considerations by Tan and Allen. Cultural sensitivity and humility topics are woven throughout this issue, a key consideration in caring for individuals with diverse backgrounds.

With a turn toward specific medical conditions, Pottie and Girard detail assessment and treatment of common infectious conditions. Brickhill-Atkinson and Hauck highlight the impact of the coronavirus pandemic on the refugee population, a timely topic for this issue. DiVito and colleagues provide an overview of common medical conditions affecting refugees, immigrants, and asylees. Payton and colleagues detail preventive care for adults, while Simha and Brown provide specific and relevant recommendations for comprehensive care of pediatric patients. Turn to the article by Huffstetler and coauthors for a complete guide to women's health care; the authors detail comprehensive care in the context of a woman's prior experiences with health care and beliefs about health. Griswold and colleagues address the critical topic of mental health care in refugees and immigrants with a scoping article focused on diagnostic and treatment considerations. Complexity is a hallmark of refugee care, as described in a series of cases by Johnson and colleagues, who also highlight the importance of attention to social determinants of health and the role of the medical community in advocating for refugees.

Perhaps, with the knowledge gained from this issue, your interest in caring for refugees, immigrants, and asylees will be ignited—or reignited! If that is the case, turn to the article by Elmore and colleagues—the authors comprehensively identify key features of successful clinics providing full-scope primary care to refugees, immigrants, and asylees. In caring for these individuals, you may find yourself challenged in new ways with new clinical questions. We hope within this issue you find the answers as you seek to provide exceptional care for these vulnerable populations.

Fern R. Hauck, MD, MS, FAAFP
Department of Family Medicine
University of Virginia
PO Box 800729
Charlottesville, VA 22908-0729, USA

Carina M. Brown, MD
Cone Health Family Medicine Residency
UNC-Chapel Hill
Department of Family Medicine
1125 North Church Street
Greensboro, NC 27284, USA

E-mail addresses:
frh8e@virginia.edu (F.R. Hauck)
Carina.brown@conehealth.com (C.M. Brown)

Caring for the Forcibly Displaced

Jeffrey Walden, MD

KEYWORDS

- Refugee • Immigrant • Migrants

KEY POINTS

- The number of those forcibly displaced from their home countries continues to rise, while the number of nations accepting these peoples for resettlement continues to downtrend.
- Resettled refugees do not enter their destination country until they have legal admittance obtained while still overseas, whereas asylees apply for protected status once they reach their destination country.
- The vetting process for intake of new refugees arriving in the United States is both stringent and detailed, and can take upward of 36 months.
- Refugees and other immigrants often face various difficulties obtaining adequate health care after arrival in their destination countries.

BACKGROUND AND TRENDS

Due to changing political landscapes both in the United States and worldwide, immigration and refugee issues remain much in the news, with little indication that these issues will be resolved in the near future. Presently there are more displaced people worldwide than at any point in history. That number first reached a historic high in 2015 with 65 million displaced people, the most since World War II.[1] The number has only increased since that time. In 2019, we reached an unprecedented 68.5 million displaced people throughout the world according to the United Nations High Commissioner for Refugees (UNHCR).[2] Roughly one-third of those displaced have crossed international borders while fleeing persecution and violence and thereby have been labeled refugees.

Although immigration terms are often used interchangeably, there are notable differences between designations. Starting in the 1930s and 1940s, and as a consequence of Jewish persons fleeing persecution from Nazi Germany, the international community began working on an international classification for those fleeing persecution. Formal codification came in 1951 with the Convention Relating to the Status of Refugees. Based on this legal framework, a refugee is defined as someone who, "owing to

Department of Family Medicine, University of Montana, 401 Railroad Street West, Missoula, MT 59802, USA
E-mail address: jeff.walden@mso.umt.edu

Prim Care Clin Office Pract 48 (2021) 1–7
https://doi.org/10.1016/j.pop.2020.11.001
0095-4543/21/© 2020 Elsevier Inc. All rights reserved.

a well-founded fear of being persecuted for reasons of race, religion, nationality, membership of a particular social group or political opinion, is outside the country of his nationality and is unable or, owing to such fear, is unwilling to avail himself of the protection of that country."[3]

DEFINITIONS

Definitions remain important when discussing newcomers arriving in the United States, especially as pertaining to health care matters. The US immigration system uses particular language when dealing with specific types of immigrants. Many times, however, these terms may be used interchangeably by politicians or those in the press. As mentioned previously, the 1951 international classification defines refugees as those fleeing some form of persecution while outside their home country. Those found to meet these qualifications, and who cannot be returned to their home countries or integrated into their host country, are then referred for resettlement into a third nation. If referred to the United States, before admission, refugee applicants are processed overseas first by officials with the UNHCR and then numerous US federal agencies, resulting in a vetting process that can take up to 24 months.[4] Refugee status is therefore not automatically granted but determined only after this vetting process. All refugees who have arrived in the United States have thereby done so through this legal channel.

Newcomers who proclaim political asylum, however, are those who state they meet the qualifications for being a refugee but "but whose claim has not yet been definitively evaluated."[5] Similar to refugees, those seeking political asylum are outside their home nation, and often seek asylum in their destination country. The validity of the claims for those seeking political asylum, therefore, have yet to be determined, and individuals must process their claims through the federal immigration court system. The term "immigrant" generally exists as a blanket term or catch-all for those outside of their country of origin. Such newcomers often are also seeking permanent residence, but have left their home countries for opportunities such as work, education, or for family reunification.[6] That said, many immigrants have also witnessed or experienced violence in their home countries, but otherwise do not meet the criteria for either refugee or asylum status. As a final note, immigrants may or may not have documentation authorizing their residence in the United States.

Since 1975, the United States has resettled approximately 3 million refugees total,[7] and an average number between 70,000 and 80,000 refugees per year, with a steep drop-off in the past several years because of changes instituted by the Trump administration,[8] followed by Canada with approximately 658,000 refugees resettled and Australia at 486,000.[9] As of 2018, Canada has resettled more refugees per year than the United States, making it the top nation for resettled refugees.[10] Canada resettled 28,100 refugees, followed by the United States (22,900), Australia (12,700), the United Kingdom (5800), and France (5600)[10]; 2018 marked the first year the United States was not the top refugee resettlement nation since the adoption of the Refugee Act in 1980. This downtrend in acceptance was preceded by 2017, which was the first year the United States had not resettled more refugees than the entire rest of the world combined.[10] The US trends both highlight and directly contribute to resettlement trends worldwide. Globally, trends reveal a continued and marked decrease in refugee resettlement. In 2018, 92,000 refugees were resettled, as opposed to 103,000 in 2017 and 189,000 in 2016.[10]

With almost 30 million refugees worldwide, these numbers mean less than 0.3% of the world's refugees are resettled in any given year. Despite nativist concerns over increased migration patterns, these numbers mean that as a nation, the United States, as well as other resettlement nations, can thereby exercise much discretion when selecting which refugees enter the country. Indeed, the process to vet potential refugees involves security clearances by numerous federal agencies, including the Department of Homeland Security, and can take upward of 18 to 36 months.

SCREENING AND EVALUATIONS

Those who have applied for either refugee status specifically or immigrant visas more generally must undergo a medical examination while still overseas and before admission to the United States.[11] Performed by panel physicians, these health care workers use Centers for Disease Control and Prevention (CDC)-established guidelines to identify any medical condition that would pose a significant public health danger to the United States.[12] After arrival in the United States, the CDC recommends, and some states mandate, that newly arrived refugees undergo a domestic screening evaluation based on further CDC guidelines.[11] Not all newcomers are refugees, and therefore health care workers at all levels should be vigilant and ensure all newcomers receive appropriate care. See Kelly Reese and Brianna Moyer's article, "Refugee Medical Screening," in this issue, for more details of the overseas and domestic examinations.

For refugees specifically, after arrival in the United States, individuals or families are matched with a voluntary resettlement agency, otherwise known as a Volag. These Volags are tasked with coordinating placement within communities based on host community readiness, available services, and housing opportunities.[13] Refugees receive assistance applying for a Social Security number, enrolling any children in school, enrolling in English language classes, and seeking employment opportunities. Refugees also receive government cash assistance and medical assistance, although these are limited to the first 8 months after arrival, as refugees are expected to be self-sufficient after that period.

Historically, the United States has not discriminated on a refugee's case based on his or her ability to integrate. Although this ensures granting the most vulnerable equal access to protection and resettlement, refugees therefore often arrive with untreated or even undiagnosed chronic or serious health problems. Existing protocols allow for initial screening and evaluation of those undergoing migration both domestically and abroad. However, after arrival in the United States, many newcomers face access to care difficulties that extend far beyond the initial screening. Furthermore, many of these newcomers may have experienced persecution and trauma at the hands of government officials previously, especially if the newcomers are refugees, and therefore they may be more hesitant to seek care because of an inherent distrust of those in positions of authority.[14]

Beyond just health care issues, immigrants and refugees also face other difficulties when trying to integrate into a new society, including transportation issues and inabilities to access interpretation resources when attempting to engage medical, dental, or mental health facilities.[15] Acculturation stress can negatively impact those who wind up outside of their country of origin. Although refugees have risk factors for mental health disorders, by definition of their prior traumas, other immigrants have been thought to benefit from what has been termed "the healthy migrant affect." Attempting to navigate a particularly bureaucratic process, namely documented immigration, often eliminates all but those best educated or most resilient. However, the data behind this effect is weak; indeed, the health status of immigrants often worsens after migration.[16,17]

BEHIND THE NUMBERS

And yet, in spite of the resources provided to refugees or the inherent health effects of immigrants, and despite the ongoing political challenges to newcomers arriving in the United States as evidenced by decreasing arrivals, the preceding numbers remain just that: numbers. What can be lost in statistics are the images and stories of those who undergo lives of forced migration. Those of us who have spent years working with these groups have numerous stories to tell. Allow one couple to serve as an example. Although details have been changed to protect confidentiality, the essence of the story remains.

Picture a young couple, husband and wife, originally from a small country in East Africa, who fell in love despite being members of separate tribal families. The couple met and began seeing each other while attempting to hide their courtship. Yet theirs was a small village, and word of their being together eventually got out. The woman had several brothers, and 1 day these brothers met the man after he was leaving his job. The man worked as an auto mechanic, and the brothers used several of his tools to severely beat him. The assault served as a warning to discourage any further attempts to meet with their sister. The man awoke in a pool of his own blood and eventually crawled back home.

The brothers didn't stop there. They drove home and told their sister what they had done. When she protested, they beat her as well and threatened to lock her up in the house so she could never leave to meet him.

She escaped several days later, never to see her family again. The woman ran to her love and helped him recover, and once he was well enough to travel, they fled into the bush where they lived with a family friend in hiding for almost a year. The husband worked small, odd jobs during this time to support the 2 of them. They also married.

The 2 remained in hiding, yet even so, the man eventually heard whispers that the brothers were looking for them to kill them. He knew they could not stay, and to his mind there was only one place that would truly be safe, and thus he began searching for a way to make it to America.

For several weeks, he set about, as circumspectly as possible, inquiring ways to travel to safety. Through his boss, he learned of a ship captain who would stow away the man and his wife for a small fee. They were promised passage for only a portion of their trip, and they were not told where they would be going. They had 1 day to make their decision, as the ship left the following morning.

By this time, the woman was several months pregnant. So they faced a choice: stay in their own country, the only land they had known, where they knew the monetary system, the local politics, the language, their friends, yet risk likely death if discovered. Or, they could leave their home, board a ship, travel to an unknown land under protection of a captain they had not met, and then have to make the rest of their way on their own. All with the wife being pregnant.

They chose the ship. They met the captain the next day and stowed away in the ship's cargo hold, near the engines, a section of the vessel that had no climate control. They roasted during the day and clung together for warmth against the chill at night. The shrieks and groans of the engines through the walls kept them awake at all hours of the day. They were brought one meal each day and a single pitcher of water, but as the journey continued, the wife became deathly seasick, to the point she became unable to tolerate even the smallest meals. Knowing she needed medicine and had become dehydrated from the constant vomiting, the husband risked detection and left the cargo hold. He found several workers and explained their situation. Luck was on his side, and they brought his wife medicine and more water. She remained weak through the trip, but could manage.

When they finally landed 10 days later, the ship captain wished them well, and they found themselves in a land where, despite speaking a total of 8 languages between them, they could not understand a thing anyone said in this new country. All they knew was that they had to travel north as fast as possible before what little money they still had ran out. As the husband made inquiries at the local bus depot, he finally found someone who spoke English, and learned they had landed in Colombia, South America. They bought 2 bus tickets and boarded a bus north that night.

They continued north on that same bus through Central America, the pregnant wife remaining ill for much of the journey and the husband distraught because they did not have enough money to seek care for her, before they finally arrived at the border town of Tijuana, just south of San Diego. When they attempted to cross the border, they were found to have no legal documentation, and placed in detention. While in detention, they claimed asylum, asking not to be returned to their home country.

Asylum is an ancient judicial concept, and modern political asylum is a legal right granted to those who have fled their home country due to risk of persecution, similar to refugee status, as mentioned previously. It is critical to remember that those seeking asylum in the United States do not simply seek a better job or better opportunities for themselves and their families. These are people who, if returned to their home countries, risk persecution, torture, and death. They are here out of fear.

While awaiting trial for asylum, you are not a citizen. You are unable to work, receive no benefits, have no health insurance, receive no supplemental support. Asylees in the United States generally endure this difficult time being taken in by religious or other social organizations. The average time to process an asylum's claim through immigration court is 721 days (almost 2 years), although at times it can be far longer.[18]

After potential asylees obtain an immigration attorney, the attorney will most likely request a medical forensic evaluation. This assumes the client is able to obtain an immigration attorney; most attorneys charge fees, and one can imagine the difficulties this poses for people unable to work. The purpose of the medical forensic evaluation is to examine a client to ascertain any history of torture via either a physical or psychological evaluation. An entire field of science exists around the study of torture and what human beings have contrived to do to one another. For those clients who do not obtain a medical examination, only 37% of the cases are granted asylum. For those who do, that number jumps to 90%.[19]

Thus did the couple find themselves thousands of miles from their home country, sitting in a family medicine clinic, explaining their story and revealing their scars, both physical and mental.

CURRENT CHALLENGES

Such stories are, unfortunately, not uncommon. And yet it can be that, within the walls of a medical clinic, hospital, or other health care setting, individuals finally allow themselves the opportunity to open up about their past. Clinicians can provide a level of trust and security for newcomer patients that might otherwise be lacking in society today. This is the basis for this issue and the following articles. No matter your interest in immigrant health, you will be able to find answers to what you are seeking here, and hopefully you will feel more heartened to see newcomer populations, in whatever clinical setting you work.

Finally, a word of caution: those of us who are able to listen, who find ourselves involved in such work, also concurrently find ourselves overwhelmed, disheartened, and sometimes burned out. The challenges of working with these populations are vast, and resources—time, money, political assurances—diminishing. Many of those who care for newcomer populations have been doing so for years, if not decades, and were doing so long before recent political changes elevated the health and welfare of immigrants and refugees to society's forefront. Others have become interested in immigrant health precisely because of this increased focus. This is likely a good thing; the causes of migration—ongoing warfare, environmental changes, populist concerns—are not likely ending anytime soon. Each group will need the other in the challenging times ahead: new energy and experience working together.

DISCLOSURE

The author has nothing to disclose.

REFERENCES

1. The Office of the United Nations High Commissioner for Refugees. Global trends: forced displacement in 2015. Geneva (Switzerland): UNCHR; 2016. Available at: https://www.unhcr.org/576408cd7. Accessed May 20, 2020.
2. The Office of the United Nations High Commissioner for Refugees Figures at a Glance. UNCHR website. Available at: https://www.unhcr.org/figures-at-a-glance.html. Accessed May 20, 2020.
3. The Office of the United Nations High Commissioner for Refugees. The 1951 Refugee Convention. UNCHR Web site. Available at: http://www.unhcr.org/pages/49da0e466.html. Accessed May 19, 2020.
4. US Department of State. U.S. Refugee Admissions Program: application and case processing. US Department of State Web site. Available at: http://www.state.gov/j/prm/ra/admissions. Accessed May 17, 2020.
5. The Office of the United Nations High Commissioner for Refugees Asylum-Seekers. UNCHR Web site. Available at: http://www.unhcr.org/pages/49c3646c137.html. Accessed May 19, 2020.
6. U.S. Citizenship and Immigration Services Lawful Permanent Resident. USCIS Web site. Available at: https://www.uscis.gov/tools/glossary/lawful-permanent-resident. Accessed May 14, 2020.
7. Igielnik R, Krogstad JM. Where refugees to the U.S. come from. Pew Research Web site. Available at: http://www.pewre-search.org/fact-tank/2017/02/03/where-refugees-to-the-u-s-come-from/. Accessed February 3, 2020.
8. Migration Policy Institute U.S. Annual Refugee Resettlement Ceilings and Numbers of Refugees Admitted, 1980-Present. Migration Policy Institute Web site. Available at: https://www.migrationpolicy.org/programs/data-hub/charts/us-annual-refugee-resettlement-ceilings-and-number-refugees-admitted-united. Accessed January 29, 2020.
9. Canada now leads the world in refugee resettlement, surpassing the US. Pew Research Center Web site. Available at: https://www.pewresearch.org/fact-tank/2019/06/19/canada-now-leads-the-world-in-refugee-resettlement-surpassing-the-u-s/?utm_source=AdaptiveMailer&utm_medium=email&utm_campaign=6-19-19%20Refugee%20Resettlement%20Post&org=982&lvl=100&ite=4235&lea=979527&ctr=0&par=1&trk=. Accessed August 13, 2020.
10. Global Trends forced displacement in 2018. UNHCR Web site. Available at: https://www.unhcr.org/statistics/unhcrstats/5d08d7ee7/unhcr-global-trends-2018.html. Accessed August 13, 2020.
11. Refugee health guidelines: guidelines for pre-departure and post-arrival medical screening and treatment of U.S.-bound refugees. CDC Web site. 2013. Available

at: http://www.cdc.gov/immigrantrefugeehealth/guidelines/refugee-guidelines. html. November 12. Accessed April 20, 2020.

12. Rew KT, Clarke SL, Gossa W, et al. Immigrant and refugee health: medical evaluation. FP Essent 2014;423:11–8.
13. Walden J, Valdman O, Mishori R, et al. Building capacity to care for refugees. Fam Pract Manag 2017;24(4):21–7.
14. Pereira KM, Crosnoe R, Fortuny K, et al. Office of the Assistant Secretary for Planning and Evaluation Barriers to immigrants' access to health and human services programs. 2012. Available at: https://aspe.hhs.gov/basic-report/barriers-immigrants-access-health-and-human-services-programs. Accessed May 14, 2020.
15. Walden J, Sienkiewicz H. Immigrant and refugee health in North Carolina. N C Med J 2019;80(2):84–8.
16. Rubalcava LN, Teruel GM, Thomas D, et al. The healthy migrant effect: new findings from the Mexican Family Life Survey. Am J Public Health 2008;98(1):78–84.
17. Antecol H, Bedard K. Unhealthy assimilation: why do immigrants converge to American health status levels? Demography 2006;43(2):337–60.
18. Fact Sheet: US Asylum Process. 2019. Available at: https://immigrationforum.org/article/fact-sheet-u-s-asylum-process. Accessed June 1, 2020.
19. Lustig SL, Kureshi S, Delucchi KL, et al. Asylum grant rates following medical evaluations of maltreatment among political asylum applicants in the United States. J Immigr Minor Health 2008;10(1):7–15.

Refugee Medical Screening

Kelly Reese, MD*, Brianna Moyer, MD

KEYWORDS

- Domestic medical screening • Immunizations • Health conditions • Refugees
- Immigrants

KEY POINTS

- Refugees have a screening examination completed 6 months before departure from their host country.
- Initial domestic medical screening is a comprehensive medical and mental health visit that should include screening for infectious diseases, chronic medical conditions, and mental health concerns, addressing contraceptive management, updating immunizations, and introducing preventive health topics.
- Common medical conditions that may be encountered during the domestic medical screening examination include latent tuberculosis infection, hepatitis B, parasitic infections, eosinophilia, and micronutrient deficiencies.

Domestic medical screening of refugees is an important step for refugees coming to the United States. They come into the encounter with a great deal of insecurity, and although they are eager to prove their worthiness, they may also have genuine health concerns that have long gone unaddressed. The first health care encounter can set them up for failure or success in future interactions with health care, so it is important to provide this care in a culturally sensitive way and in a language that they understand. It is also important to quickly identify any medical conditions of public health significance. The medical screening is a time to test for infectious diseases, identify chronic medical conditions, update required vaccines, screen for mental health issues, introduce health maintenance topics, and establish a plan for reproductive health. The medical screening examination contains many elements, so it is imperative to be prepared and to devote enough time to the visit. As the first interaction with a new medical system, it establishes an important tone for a refugee's future health care. This manuscript primarily focuses on the overseas and domestic screening examination process for refugees; additional guidelines for immigrants and asylees can be found through the Centers for Disease Control and Prevention (CDC) and Physicians for Human Rights.[1,2]

Family & Community Medicine Residency Program, Penn Medicine Lancaster General Health, 540 North Duke Street, Lancaster, PA 17602, USA
* Corresponding author.
E-mail address: Kelly.Reese2@pennmedicine.upenn.edu

Prim Care Clin Office Pract 48 (2021) 9–21
https://doi.org/10.1016/j.pop.2020.09.003

MEDICAL SCREENING BEFORE DEPARTURE FROM HOST COUNTRY
Overseas Medical Screening of Refugees

A medical screening examination is required for all refugees before admission to the United States (**Fig. 1**). These examinations are done in the host country by panel physicians selected and certified by the Department of State.[2] They are completed approximately 6 months before the scheduled departure. This examination is done to identify any class A medical or behavioral health issues that would exclude a refugee from admission to the United States and to identify chronic conditions that might affect a refugee's safety during travel. The CDC maintains a list of Communicable Diseases of Public Health Significance. Currently this list includes active tuberculosis (TB), syphilis, gonorrhea, and Hansen disease (leprosy). Substance use disorder is also a class A condition. Human immunodeficiency virus (HIV) is no longer a disease that precludes admission to the United States and is not a required predeparture test. Quarantinable diseases designated by any Presidential order will also exclude a refugee from admission. Class B conditions are medical or mental health conditions that do not preclude admission to the United States but may interfere with activities of daily living or require ongoing monitoring or treatment.[3]

Tuberculosis Screening

All refugees older than 2 years are screened for TB.[4] Applicants 2 through 14 years of age are screened for TB based on medical history (including a survey of symptoms such as cough of greater than 3-week duration, fever, weight loss, night sweats, and hemoptysis), family medical history of TB and physical examination. Those living in a country with an incidence greater than or equal to 20 cases per 100,000 population undergo an interferon gamma release assay (IGRA) test. Any positive result prompts a chest radiograph for further evaluation. If the chest radiograph is abnormal, 3 sputum samples are collected for smear and culture. Applicants 15 years of age and older from all countries (regardless of incidence of TB) are tested for TB with a history, physical examination, and a screening chest radiograph. If the radiograph is

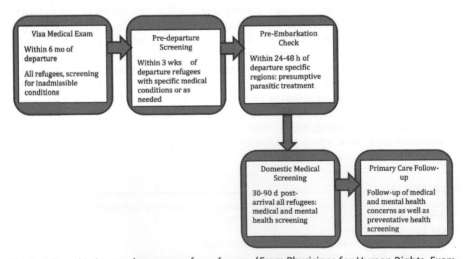

Fig. 1. US medical screening process for refugees. (*From* Physicians for Human Rights. Examining asylum seekers: A clinician's guide to physical and psychological evaluations of torture and ill-treatment. Cambridge, MA: Physicians for Human Rights; 2012; with permission.)

suspicious for active or previous TB, 3 sputum samples are collected and smears and cultures for TB completed. For all age groups, if the sputum is positive, the patient is treated for active TB according to susceptibility data from the sputum culture. After completion of treatment, repeat sputum samples are obtained to demonstrate cure before a refugee can be cleared for immigration. Prior receipt of BCG vaccine will not affect the results of the IGRA. Refugees with positive IGRA and negative chest radiograph or abnormal chest radiograph with negative sputum samples can be cleared for immigration but will need follow-up treatment of latent TB on arrival in the United States. Latent TB is not a diagnosis for exclusion from immigration.

Hepatitis B Screening

Refugees are tested for hepatitis B with a surface antigen test if they come from an area that is participating in the Vaccination Program for US-bound refugees. Test results are noted on their overseas medical record.[5]

Immunizations

Adult refugees are usually immunized for tetanus and diphtheria with a Td (tetanus and diphtheria) vaccine. They usually get 2 doses of this vaccine before departure.[5] They also usually get at least 2 doses of MMR (measles, mumps, and rubella) vaccine if they were born in or after 1957. If they were born before 1957, they can be presumed to have natural immunity, and vaccination is not indicated. More doses of the individual components of the MMR vaccine might be given for local outbreaks.[6] Although polio has been eradicated in the United States, there are still cases of wild poliovirus infection as well as vaccine-derived poliovirus infection around the globe. Immigrants who have spent 4 weeks or more in the past year in countries with ongoing outbreaks (Afghanistan, Pakistan, Nigeria, Indonesia, Malaysia, Myanmar, and Philippines) should have a bivalent oral polio vaccine or inactivated polio vaccine given in the 12 months before they come to the United States.[7] Children may get age-appropriate vaccines depending on the recommendations of their home country. Vaccines listed on the overseas medical record are in the format of day-month (3-letter abbreviation for month)-year.

Overseas Presumptive Treatment

Refugees are given presumptive treatment of parasites such as soil helminths, schistosomiasis, and malaria 1 to 2 days before departure from their country of origin depending on recommendations for the host country. The usual treatments are albendazole and ivermectin for soil helminths, praziquantel for schistosomiasis, and artemether-lumefantrine for malaria. Ivermectin is not given to refugees from The Democratic Republic of Congo and South Sudan because *Loa loa* is endemic to these areas; treatment with ivermectin in these cases can cause serious adverse events.[8] Presumptive treatment is not given to pregnant women or to children younger than 1 year.

DOMESTIC MEDICAL SCREENINGS

Refugees are required to have a medical screening examination including laboratory evaluation within 30 to 90 days of their arrival in the United States. There are elements of this medical examination that are common to any new patient encounter, but there are also parts that are unique to refugee health care. The CDC provides guidance for testing, and individual states may have their own additional requirements for testing. An excellent resource is provided by a Web site curated by the Minnesota Department of Health and Minnesota Center for Excellence in Refugee Health that lists the local health alerts for the country of origin and the state-specific recommended screening tests and procedures once the specific demographics of the refugee are entered.[9] There are required vaccines for school and for lawful permanent resident applications. These vaccine series are begun or completed during the domestic medical screening examination depending on serologies and previously documented vaccines. Any vaccines that were given overseas are valid as long as they are given at an appropriate age and interval. Refugees should bring a copy of their overseas medical examination with them or the resettlement agency may provide it. This will include a physical examination; documentation of screening for active TB; a list of medications and medical conditions; vaccine records; and a record of predeparture treatments for soil helminths, schistosomiasis, and malaria. If they do not have this with them, it can be accessed via the EDN (the CDC's Electronic Disease Notification system). Access to this site is restricted but can be arranged for a health care provider by the local state refugee resettlement coordinator.

Travel History

It is important to obtain a thorough travel history, as this can affect the infectious diseases that refugees have been exposed to as well as the trauma that they might have experienced. This information should be explored in a culturally sensitive way, and it should be clear that this information will not affect a refugee's resettlement status.

Family Medical History

This information is as helpful for refugees as it is for other groups but is often unknown as family members may have passed away from undiagnosed infectious disease or trauma or may have been separated after departure from the home country. Eliciting this information can be potentially traumatizing so care should be taken in exploring this information. It is helpful to see family units together if possible so that cases of hepatitis, HIV, and TB can be linked.

Refugee Health Profiles

The CDC collects information about specific refugee groups in order to improve care provided to them specifically. This information includes health concerns that are unique to that particular group, demographics, and background information.[10] Having an understanding of this information for refugee groups can help clinicians better serve refugees as individuals.

Mental Health Screen

Screening for mental illness is an important part of the initial domestic medical screening given the increased prevalence of posttraumatic stress disorder (PTSD) and depression in the refugee population.[11] Refugees are often exposed to significant stressors before resettlement. These include, but are not limited to, violence in their home country and during their journey to the host country, loss of social structures, food insecurity, housing insecurity, threats of violence in the refugee camps, domestic violence, gender-based violence, and conscription as child soldiers. Refugees resettled in Western countries may be up to 10 times more likely to have PTSD than the age-matched general population in those countries.[11] The CDC recommends screening for depression and PTSD at the initial medical screening for all refugees older than 16 years.[12] The Patient Health Questionnaire-9 and the Refugee Health Screener-15 are screening tools for depression that have been studied in a variety of cultural groups and refugee populations, respectively.[13] The CDC recommends the Posttraumatic Stress Disorder (PTSD) Checklist—Civilian version or the PTSD portion of the Harvard Trauma Questionnaire as screening tools for symptoms of PTSD in the refugee population.[12] The purpose of screening on arrival is to differentiate individuals who need immediate psychiatric referral from those with less acute symptoms of mental illness. For those individuals who do not require immediate psychiatric care, the screening provider should emphasize the importance of establishing care with a primary care provider for ongoing evaluation and assessment of the individual's mental health needs.[14] There is evidence to support the use of treatment of refugees with PTSD even with the many barriers such as language and culture that might make typical counseling therapies seem awkward or time consuming.[15]

Activities of Daily Living

For refugees who are elderly or who have special needs, the initial examination is a good time to ask about activities of daily living. Information about their ability to care for themselves may become important later when they apply for additional services, so it is helpful to establish a baseline level of functioning.

Physical Examination

A full physical examination should be performed. This is likely a refugee's first encounter with the medical system in the United States, and it may be their first encounter with some of the technology that is used in a medical encounter. Refugees are often not accustomed to many of the procedural parts of the visit that are common in the US medical system. Even simple things as the use of the examination table may require some amount of explanation.

Common findings on physical examination

- Vital sign abnormalities reflective of anxiety, such as elevated blood pressure or tachycardia
- Poor dentition
- Chronic, untreated tympanic membrane perforation
- Lung examination consistent with obstructive airway disease may be related to chronic exposure to cooking fires
- Abnormal heart sounds related to untreated congenital heart disease or post-streptococcal rheumatic heart disease
- Splenomegaly, especially in the Congolese refugee population
- Musculoskeletal deformities related to poorly healed fractures, untreated congenital deformities, or dysplasia
- Skin findings related to tropical skin diseases as well as scars from prior medical procedures or trauma

Immunizations

- A primary tetanus series is required at the time of lawful permanent resident application for all age-appropriate refugees, which is usually 1 year after arrival. For adults, this includes 3 tetanus vaccines separated by 1 month between dose number 1 and number 2 and 6 months between dose number 2 and number 3. Children should follow the CDC catch-up vaccine schedule.[16]
- MMR vaccine series is required for age-appropriate refugees. The first dose is given at 1 year of life. In other countries, it is given earlier, but this dose should not be considered valid in the United States. The second dose is given after age 4 years or 1 month after the first dose in refugees older than 4 years but born in or after 1957. Refugees born before 1957 can be presumed to have

natural immunity. They do not need vaccination, and they do not need testing for immunity.[17]

- Refugees must have a current flu vaccine if they are applying for their lawful permanent residence in flu season.[16]
- Children must have documentation of childhood vaccines, complete a catch-up schedule, or demonstrate immunity to required vaccines for school admission. If there is documentation of an incomplete series, the series should be completed even if serology demonstrates immunity.
- The decision to test for serologic evidence of immunity should be made after balancing costs of the test with the likelihood of exposure to a disease, number of vaccines required to complete a series, and the cost of vaccinations.
- In refugees for whom hepatitis A vaccination would be indicated by Advisory Committee on Immunization Practices (ACIP), testing for immunity before vaccination may be cost-effective. Routine testing for hepatitis A infection is not indicated.
- Refugees who can provide a reliable oral or written history of having varicella disease do not require vaccination or serology. The reliable history must contain an epidemiologic connection to another case of typical varicella.[18]
- Children who have received pneumococcal conjugate vaccine (PCV) 10 in another country should follow recommendations similar to those who had a history of receiving PCV7. For children who are not yet finished with their primary pneumococcal vaccine series, the series should be completed with PCV13. For children aged 14 years through 59 months who have received an age-appropriate series of 10-valent PCV (PCV10), administer a single supplemental dose of 13-valent PCV (PCV13) (Personal communication, C. Robinson, CDC, December 11, 2019).
- Recommend the human papillomavirus vaccination, although this is not required.
- Immunizations given earlier than recommended by the CDC should not be considered valid and should be repeated. Immunizations should be given according to the CDC's catch up schedule for vaccines. Adults should get all age- and disease-specific vaccinations as recommended by the ACIP.[19]
- The Immunization Action Coalition provides materials to translate foreign vaccine records.[20]

COMMON HEALTH CONDITIONS ENCOUNTERED DURING THE DOMESTIC MEDICAL SCREENING EXAMINATION
Hepatitis B

The CDC recommends that all refugees who were born in or have lived in countries with an intermediate (2%–7%) or high ($\geq$8%) prevalence of chronic hepatitis B virus (HBV) infection should be screened for HBV at their initial medical screening examination.[21] Medical providers should review overseas records, as an increasing number of refugee populations are being screened for HBV as part of predeparture testing. Some refugees may receive up to 2 doses of the HBV vaccine before departure as well. If testing has not been previously completed, serum hepatitis B surface antigen, hepatitis B surface antibody, and hepatitis B core antibody should be ordered. Individuals who do not have HBV infection but are household contacts of hepatitis B positive individuals or are school age should be offered the hepatitis B vaccination series. Individuals who screen positive for HBV infection should be referred for further testing and treatment.[21] If the hepatitis B vaccine series has been started but not completed, the series should be completed regardless of serology results (**Table 1**).

Table 1
Interpretation of hepatitis B serologic testing 2121

HBsAg	HBcAb	HBsAb	Interpretation of Results
-	-	-	Never infected, susceptible to infection
+	+	-	HBV infection, further testing required to determine if acute or chronic infection
-	+	+	Immune following natural infection
-	-	+	Immune due to hepatitis B vaccination
-	+	-	Unclear interpretation, may represent a resolved infection, false positive, chronic infection with a low viral load, or a resolving acute infection

Adapted from Centers for Disease Control and Prevention (CDC). Immigrant and Refugee Health. Screening for Viral Hepatitis During the Domestic Medical Examination of Newly Arrived Refugees. Available at: https://www.cdc.gov/immigrantrefugeehealth/guidelines/domestic/hepatitis-screening-guidelines.html. Accessed June 6 2020.

Parasitic Infections

Predeparture evaluation for refugees traveling to the United States includes empirical treatment for parasites endemic to their country of origin and current residence, as previously described.[22] However, some refugees may not receive the recommended empirical treatment due to logistical issues or medical contraindications at the time of evaluation, including pregnancy. Therefore, providers performing the initial medical screening examination should be aware of which parasitic infections are endemic to a refugee's country of origin as well as the common symptoms and recommended treatment.[22] A brief overview of common parasitic infections in refugee populations is presented in **Table 2**.

Eosinophilia

Persistent eosinophilia in refugee populations is most likely secondary to parasitic infection.[23] If eosinophilia is noted at the initial medical evaluation, the provider should review whether or not the individual received empirical treatment of endemic parasitic infections before departure. If empirical treatment was not received and there is no contraindication to treatment, the provider can choose to test for endemic parasitic infections and treat based on results or treat empirically. The total eosinophil count should be repeated 3 to 6 months after treatment. If eosinophilia persists, a broader differential should be considered. Repeat parasitic testing is often warranted, as the most common causes of persistent eosinophilia in the refugee population include failed treatments of strongyloidiasis, schistosomiasis, and trichuriasis. However, nonparasitic causes such as asthma, drug allergy, eosinophilic leukemia, Hodgkin lymphoma, hyper eosinophilic syndrome, pemphigoid, pemphigus, and polyarteritis nodosa should also be considered.

Vitamin B12 Deficiency

Micronutrient deficiencies should be considered in all refugees, but Bhutanese refugees in particular have been found to have a high prevalence of vitamin B12 deficiency. DiVito and colleagues describes the appropriate evaluation and treatment in detail.

Table 2
Overview of common parasitic infections in refugee populations

Parasitic Infection	Endemic Areas	Presentation	Diagnosis	Treatment
Strongyloides	All countries, especially Southeast Asia	Often asymptomatic; only sign may be high eosinophil count May present with abdominal pain, nausea, diarrhea, constipation, and dry cough	Presumptive treatment if no contraindications *Strongyloides* IgG serology ± stool ova and parasite testing Test for *Loa loa* microfilaremia before treatment with ivermectin if from *Loa loa* endemic area	Ivermectin Adults and children: 200 µg/kg once daily x 2 d Should not be used presumptively if child is < 15 kg
Loa loa	West and Central Africa	Eye worm, Calabar swellings, or unexplained peripheral eosinophilia	Giemsa-stained thin and thick blood smear between 10 AM and 2 PM (adjusted to reflect local time at point of origin of traveler if just arrived)	Diethylcarbamazine (DEC) Treatment is complex and expert consultation should be considered
Soil-transmitted Helminth Infections *Ancylostoma duodenale* and *Necator americanus* (hookworm) *Ascaris lumbricoides* (ascariasis) *Trichuris trichiura* (whipworm)	All countries; especially areas with warm and moist climates and poor sanitation	Often asymptomatic or subclinical Hookworm: anemia, abdominal pain, diarrhea, eosinophilia, poor growth in kids Ascariasis: abdominal pain, cough, intestinal obstruction Trichuriasis: bloody stool, anemia	Presumptive treatment if no contraindications Two or more separate stool ova and parasite tests collected at least 12–24 h apart, as shedding may be intermittent	Albendazole Adults and children > 2 y: 400 mg orally as a single dose Children 12–23 mo: 200 mg orally as single dose Presumptive treatment not recommended for infant < 12 mo

| Schistosoma Species | All sub-Saharan African countries except Lesotho | Often asymptomatic or subclinical; asymptomatic eosinophilia
S mansoni infection: bowel wall pathology, liver cirrhosis, portal hypertension
S haematobium infection: dysuria, hematuria, urinary tract obstruction, renal failure, bladder cancer | Presumptive treatment if no contraindications
Schistosoma IgG serology ± testing of stool and urine for eggs and urine analysis for red blood cells
Note: previous treatment does not decrease Schistosoma IgG levels | Praziquantel
Adults and children > 4 y: 40 mg/kg orally for 1 day
Presumptive treatment not recommended for children < 4 y |

Data from Centers for Disease Control and Prevention (CDC). Immigrant and Refugee Health. Domestic Intestinal Parasite Guidelines: Presumptive Treatment and Screening for Strongyloidiasis, Infections Caused by Other Soil-Transmitted Helminths, and Schistosomiasis among Newly Arrived Refugees. Available at: https://www.cdc.gov/immigrantrefugeehealth/guidelines/domestic/intestinal-parasites-domestic.html. Accessed June 6 2020.

Splenomegaly

The International Organization for Migration noted a large number of Congolese refugees with splenomegaly during predeparture examinations at resettlement sites in Uganda in 2014. Following this report, the CDC recommended screening and empirically treating Congolese refugees for malaria and schistosomiasis before departure.[24] Ongoing investigation continues regarding the cause of splenomegaly in the Congolese population; however, hyperreactive malaria splenomegaly (HMS) syndrome is considered to be a probable cause in many cases. HMS occurs due to repeated exposure to malaria antigens, resulting in excessive immunoglobulin M production and splenic deposition that leads to splenomegaly. Therefore, Congolese refugees arriving in the United States who are presumed to have HMS should be tested for G6PD deficiency and if negative, treated with a 2-week course of primaquine. Refugees with splenomegaly on physical examination or on imaging should be cautioned about the risk of splenic rupture and counseled not to participate in contact sports.[25]

Female Genital Mutilation

The practice of female genital mutilation (FGM) or cutting is a cultural practice that most commonly occurs in parts of Africa, the Middle East, and Southeast Asia. Providers should be aware of this practice and the effect it can have on a woman's health, including increased risk of obstetric complications, dyspareunia and sexual dysfunction, urinary tract infections, and lasting psychological effects.[26] An external genital examination is a required part of the overseas medical evaluation but is often not completed. Therefore, providers performing initial medical screening examinations should consider performing an external genital examination if female genital mutilation is suspected.[27] Huffstetler and colleagues provides additional information regarding FGM.

CHRONIC AND ACUTE HEALTH CARE

Refugees should be queried about concerns they have for their own health, and these concerns should be addressed.

Contraception

Medroxyprogesterone injection is the most common contraceptive used in the refugee camps. Refugees are often due for their next injection on arrival. Overseas medical records do not usually include information about last injection. This will need to be elicited in conversation with the refugee. Some refugees will use intrauterine devices (IUDs) for contraception, and it should be noted that different countries offer IUDs that are not available for use in the United States.

Routine Health Maintenance

Refugees are often unfamiliar with the concept of routine health maintenance examinations such as Pap smears, mammograms, and colonoscopy. These concepts should be discussed with refugees as age appropriate. To overcome language and cultural barriers, it is helpful to use images or videos on the computer to demonstrate how tests will be performed. For Pap smears, showing a patient the speculum and specimen collection device can help alleviate anxiety around the testing procedure. High rates of gender-based violence across all refugee populations can add anxiety to the procedures,[28] so it is important to spend an adequate amount of time explaining the steps with an appropriate interpreter before and during the procedure. These tests should not necessarily be done during the first encounter with the health system, but the new refugee health screening examination is a good time to introduce the concepts of health maintenance and to prepare ahead for the health maintenance visit.

Dental Health

There is generally poor access to dental providers in the camps, and some habits (such as chewing betel nut) contribute to poor dental hygiene. Refugees should be provided with information about access to local dentists and should be educated on proper oral hygiene for themselves and for age-appropriate hygiene for their children. For nonpregnant adults, providers should consider referral to a low-cost or free dental clinic, as this service is not covered by Medicaid.

CLINICS CARE POINTS

- Local health alerts for a refugee's country of origin and the domestic state-specific recommended screening tests and procedures based on the demographics of the refugee should be reviewed.
- Check the University of Minnesota CareRef refugee screening tool for a complete list of recommended screening tests and other recommendations.
- Evidence shows providing mental health care is beneficial to refugees, in spite of significant barriers such as language, culture, and gender.
- Immunization series that are started but not completed should be completed regardless of the results of any titers.

DISCLOSURE

The authors have nothing to disclose.

REFERENCES

1. Physicians for Human Rights. Examining asylum seekers: a clinician's guide to physical and psychological evaluations of torture and ill-treatment. Cambridge (MA): Physicians for Human Rights; 2012.
2. Centers for Disease Control and Prevention. Panel Physicians Technical Instructions. 2017. Available at: https://www.cdc.gov/immigrantrefugeehealth/exams/ti/panel/technical-instructions-panel-physicians.html. Accessed June 5, 2020.
3. USCIS. Chapter 2 - Medical Examination and Vaccination Record. 2019. Available at: https://www.uscis.gov/policy-manual/volume-8-part-b-chapter-2. Accessed June 4, 2020.
4. Centers for Disease Control and Prevention. Tuberculosis Panel Physicians Technical Instructions. 2019. Available at: https://www.cdc.gov/immigrantrefugeehealth/exams/ti/panel/tuberculosis-panel-technical-instructions.html. Accessed June 4, 2020.
5. Centers for Disease Control and Prevention. Vaccination Program for US-Bound Refugees. US Department of Health and Human Services. 2019. Available at: https://www.cdc.gov/immigrantrefugeehealth/guidelines/overseas/interventions/immunizations-schedules.html. Accessed July 29, 2020.
6. Centers for Disease Control and Prevention. Vaccination Technical Instructions for Panel Physicians. 2017. Available at: www.cdc.gov/immigrantrefugeehealth/

22. www.cdc.gov\immigrantrefugeehealth\guidelines\domestic\intestinal-parasites-domestic.html Accessed June 5, 2020.

23. CDC Immigrant and Refugee Health - Intestinal Parasite Guidelines, 2020. Available at: https://www.cdc.gov/immigrantrefugeehealth/guidelines/domestic/intestinal-parasites-domestic/intestinal-parasites.html Accessed June 6, 2020 guideline.

24. Zambrano LD, Samson O, Prieto G, et al. Unresolved syndromic diarrhea in recently resettled congolese refugees: multiple states, 2015-2018. MMWR 2018 67(48): 1358-62.

25. Congolese Refugee Health Profile. Non-Communicable Diseases 2016. Available at: https://www.cdc.gov/immigrantrefugeehealth/profiles/congolese/health-information/non-communicable-disease.html. Accessed May 10, 2020.

26. Mishori R, Warren N, Reingold R, et al. Female genital mutilation or cutting. Am Fam Physician 2018;97(1):49-52.

27. CDC Refugee Health Guidelines. Female Genital Cutting. 2016. Available at: https://www.cdc.gov/immigrantrefugeehealth/guidelines/domestic/general/discussion/female-genital-cutting.html. Accessed May 10, 2020.

28. World Health Organization. Displaced or refugee women are at increased risk of gender-based violence. WHO. docs 2016. Available at: https://www.who.int/reproductivehealth/displaced-refugee-women-violence/en/. Accessed May 10, 2020.

Effective Communication with Refugees and Immigrants

Carina M. Brown, MD[a],*, Scott Bland, DO[b], Nadia Saif, MD, MPH[c]

KEYWORDS

- Communication • Communication barriers • Emigrants and immigrants
- Limited English proficiency • Refugees

KEY POINTS

- Refugees and immigrants have significantly higher rates of limited English proficiency (LEP) than their native-born counterparts.
- LEP has been identified as a barrier to accessing health care and achieving optimal health.
- Access to professional interpreter services increases provider and patient satisfaction, improves quality of care, and reduces errors in communication.
- Interpretation methods vary in terms of cost, patient satisfaction, and provider satisfaction; no single method is perfect for every clinical encounter.

INTRODUCTION

As classified by the United States Census Bureau, individuals more than 5 years of age who report speaking English less than very well are considered to have limited English proficiency (LEP).[1] Given continued and increasing global migration, the numbers of LEP individuals in the United States is large and growing. In 2013, 25.1 million residents in the United States were considered to have LEP.[1] Of LEP individuals, 5 million are described as native born in the United States.

Immigrants, refugees, and asylees account for much of the remainder. Immigrants differ from refugees in that immigrants tend to have higher rates of English proficiency (as high as 60%), whereas refugees have lower rates of attaining proficiency (approximately 40%) after resettlement.[1] Linguistic diversity is also increasing in Canada; in 2016, 7.6 million (21.8%) Canadians reported speaking a language other than the official languages of English and French at home.[2]

[a] Department of Family Medicine, Cone Health Family Medicine Residency, University of North Carolina-Chapel Hill, 1125 North Church Street, Greensboro, NC 27401, USA; [b] Cone Health Family Medicine Residency, 1125 North Church Street, Greensboro, NC 27401, USA; [c] University of Virginia Family Medicine Residency, PO Box 800729, Charlottesville, VA 22908, USA
* Corresponding author.
E-mail address: Carina.brown@conehealth.com

Prim Care Clin Office Pract 48 (2021) 23–34
https://doi.org/10.1016/j.pop.2020.09.004
primarycare.theclinics.com
0095-4543/21/© 2020 Elsevier Inc. All rights reserved.

The words interpretation and translation are often used interchangeably. However, in proper usage, interpretation refers to conversion of a message from one language to another orally, whereas translation refers to the written conversion of a message.[3] A qualified interpreter is an individual with a high level of proficiency in at least 2 languages and with the appropriate training and experience to interpret with skill and accuracy. Qualified interpreters must adhere to certain ethical standards. Bilingualism is 1 of the qualifications of a skilled interpreter. Without specific training as an interpreter, a bilingual individual may provide direct services in either language but would not be qualified to serve as an interpreter.[3] Effective and appropriate communication with LEP patients includes the use of qualified interpreters as well as preparation and education of the clinicians caring for these patients.

Health Disparities Among Patients with Limited English Proficiency

Studies show that a multitude of health disparities exist among patients with LEP compared with English-proficient patients. LEP individuals have lower rates of health insurance and are less likely to receive high-quality health care.[4] Refugees disproportionately have poor health outcomes because of several structural barriers, one of the largest of which is language.[5] Among immigrants, LEP has been identified as critical source of disparate health outcomes.[6] A 2015 study using nationally representative data found that individuals with LEP, compared with their English-proficient peers, were less likely to report that their doctors always listened carefully to them, showed respect for what they had to say, and explained things so that they could understand.[4] Data also show that language barriers can be dangerous and contribute to disparities in patient safety between LEP and English-proficient patients. The Joint Commission's Sentinel Event Database shows that communication problems are the most frequent root cause of serious patient safety events reported.[7]

The growing diversity of the patient population presents unique challenges, as well as opportunities, to health care providers. Effective communication is at the heart of patient-centered care. Widespread access to qualified language interpretation resources is paramount to tackling the disparities mentioned earlier between LEP and English-proficient patients.

Legal Requirements for Interpretation

In the United States, legislation explicitly requires provision of interpretation services for LEP patients by certain covered entities. Title VI of the Civil Rights Act of 1964 prohibits discrimination based on race, color, and national origin and requires covered entities to take reasonable steps to provide meaningful access to LEP individuals.[8] The Affordable Care Act (ACA) further defined this, and section 1557 prohibits discrimination on the basis of race, color, national origin, sex, age, or disability in certain federal health programs and activities.[9] The ACA requires facilities that participate in Medicare or Medicaid, community health centers, state public health agencies receiving federal assistance, programs administered by executive agencies, or any entity established under Title I of the ACA to provide language services to LEP individuals.[9]

Clinicians should additionally document the type and numerical identifier or name of the interpreter used for each patient encounter. LEP individuals are not required to accept language assistance services. If they decline (and, for example, request that an adult friend or family member interpret for them), clinicians should document in the individual's records that services were offered and declined.[9] It is also prohibited to rely on a minor child to interpret for an adult, except in an emergency involving an imminent threat to the safety or welfare of an individual or the public where there is no qualified interpreter immediately available.[9]

In Canada, there is no legislation requiring that interpreters be provided in the health care setting, which seems to be an important factor in the variation in language services access across provinces and territories.[10] Although the Canada Health Act does not explicitly require the provision of health care interpretation services, many argue that the right to language services falls under the key principles of access and universality outlined in the act, as well as other legislation outlining the right to informed medical decision making. Similarly, The Canadian Charter of Rights and Freedoms, the Canadian Human Rights Act, and the Canadian Multiculturalism Act have provisions for nondiscrimination, which many argue implicitly makes the case for access to language services in health care settings.[10]

Ethical Obligations for Interpretation

The National Council on Interpreting in Health Care (NCIHC) is a US-based multidisciplinary organization made up of clinicians, researchers, and interpreters whose mission is to promote and enhance language access in health care.[3] The NCIHC developed a National Code of Ethics for Interpreters in Health Care.[11] This code of ethics is founded on 3 core values:

- Beneficence: shared with other health professions, the obligation to support the health and well-being of the patient and to do no harm
- Fidelity: remaining faithful to the original message without adding to, omitting from, or distorting it
- Respect for importance of culture and cultural differences: being cognizant of and able to alert both the patient and the provider to the impact of culture in the health care encounter

National Standards for Culturally and Linguistically Appropriate Services

The US Department of Health and Human Services (DHHS) Office of Minority Health developed the National Standards for Culturally and Linguistically Appropriate Services in Health and Health Care (the National CLAS Standards). These standards outline action steps for health care systems to take to provide culturally and linguistically appropriate services, in an effort to advance health equity, improve quality, and help eliminate health disparities.[12] The blueprint, available on the CLAS Web site, offers a detailed overview of each of the standards and practical information on how to implement them in an organization.[13] The standards provide structure and guidance to establish equitable language services to LEP patients, which should include leadership dedicated to health equity and ongoing assessment of the language program. In addition, the standards state services should be offered for language and communication at no cost to patients.

Requirements for Print Materials

Rates of literacy in native languages differ considerably between immigrants, refugees, and asylees. Immigrants tend to have much higher rates of literacy and higher educational attainment compared with refugees.[14,15] Within refugee populations, rates of literacy vary considerably. For example, Laotian Hmong have a literacy rate of approximately 18%, whereas Cuban, Vietnamese, and Iraqi refugees have literacy rates higher than 75%.[14] In addition, rates of literacy vary considerably depending on the availability of education during the time of displacement and several other factors.

The National CLAS Standards state that print materials, signage, and multimedia should be published in common languages in the service area with easy-to-read print.[12] Similarly, Title VI of the Civil Rights Act applies to document translation and

Section 1557 of the ACA mandates reasonable steps be taken to provide language-concordant written materials.[8,9] To be in compliance with Title VI, covered entities must provide written notice to LEP individuals of their right to language assistance services, such as through provision of language identification (so-called I-speak cards) or signs in waiting rooms/receptions areas. Covered entities should provide translated written materials in the most frequently encountered languages (determined by the percentage of the population the LEP group constitutes), particularly of vital documents such as consent forms, applications, and notices pertaining to change in benefits or services.[8] However, because federally funded programs have unique characteristics and circumstances, the Office of Civil Rights determines a covered entity's specific obligations for translation of written materials on a case-by-case basis, taking into account several factors.[8]

TYPES OF INTERPRETERS AND COMPARISONS

There are multiple methods of interpretation that clinicians and medical staff can use to communicate with language-discordant patients.[16] In areas with higher concentrations of patients with certain native languages, many health care systems use in-person interpreters. Remote professional interpreter services provide telephonic or video services at the point of care and are readily available for many clinicians. Some patients present with a family member or friend who has more familiarity with English than the patient, termed ad hoc interpreters.

Decision making and implementation of the preferred interpretation services is a complex issue requiring stakeholder input and evaluation. Patients vary in their language skills and may differ in the frequency of use of interpreter services, which may depend on the type and complexity of the clinical situation.[17] Although patient autonomy is an important consideration, it should also be noted that both lack of access and potentially inaccurate self-assessment of need for interpretation services contribute to the documented health disparities for LEP patients.[18] Recognizing the difficulties faced by LEP patients, current National CLAS Standards indicate that all patients should be offered professional language services, both verbally and in writing, in the preferred language.[12]

Because health communication with patients encompasses more than direct physician-to-patient discussions, some health care systems have implemented more comprehensive services. One such program is the Peer Language Navigator (PLN) program developed by the Anchorage Health Literacy Collaborative.[16] The PLN program functions as a comprehensive service that teaches foreign language speakers the basic English language health and medical terms in order to serve as health literacy ambassadors to their respective language groups. Educating independent health literacy ambassadors, such as the Anchorage PLN program, allows improvements in community health knowledge without placing 1:1 time restraints on clinicians.[16] These programs can be force multipliers in improving health literacy as well as developing relationships between a health system and an at-risk group.

Comparative Efficacy

In-person interpretation is the most traditional form of professional medical interpretation. Availability of these highly trained individuals is often limited by distance and cost. In areas with a high concentration of language groups, in-person interpretation can more easily be provided. Providers often prefer this method of interpretation.[19] Patients may not prefer this method, particularly for sensitive examinations.[19] In addition, in some close-knit communities, the interpreter and patient may frequently be in contact outside of the health care setting. Permission should be obtained from the patient to use an in-person interpreter.

Live video interpretation, preferably on larger screens, allows the interpreter to visualize hand gestures, motions, and facial expressions. Video may result in a higher degree of accuracy in interpretation and a lower error and repetition rate. Compared with telephone services, video interpreter services seem to result in higher rates of patient comprehension and have fewer lapses in interpretation.[20] High resolution is necessary for accurate interpretation for patients with hearing impairment. The video screen should be positioned such that the interpreter can see the patient for most of the encounter. During sensitive portions of the examination, to protect privacy, the video screen can be rotated or turned off such that the interpreter cannot see the patient.

Telephone interpreters offer the benefit of standard of training and easy, quick access to many languages.[19] However, nonverbal cues in the patient's expression and mood can be missed as well as body language that might be culturally significant. For some patients wishing to discuss issues that might be sensitive or embarrassing in their culture, the impersonal nature of a telephone interpreter can be preferable.

Ad hoc interpreters have the benefit of being known and trusted by the patient. Although there may be a perceived benefit in honoring patient autonomy and potential comfort level, errors in translation by ad hoc interpreters are more likely to be clinically significant.[21] In some cases, the interpreter's close relationship with the patient might inhibit the patient's willingness to share information that can be considered confidential or culturally sensitive, particularly if a young adult child is serving as the interpreter for the encounter. Professional interpreter services should always be offered first and recommended.

Bilingual clinicians require special consideration as interpreters. This option was previously thought to be the gold standard of interpretative services, although many now consider in-person professionally trained interpreters to be the gold standard with which other forms are compared. Patients may be less satisfied with bilingual clinicians acting as interpreters in clinical settings.[19] Bilingual staff and clinicians should undergo proficiency assessment before providing interpretation services to their patients.

Professional interpreter services improve patient satisfaction, increase quality of care, and reduce health care use.[22] Multiple studies have compared different formats of interpretation in a variety of clinical areas (**Fig. 1**).[19,20,23] Providers generally prefer in-person interpreter services. Some data show a reduction in the total duration of emergency department visits with in-person interpretation services. Other data show that providers spend less time speaking with patients when telephone interpreter services are used compared with video or in-person services.[23] These findings raise the concern for incomplete assessment and potential for diagnostic error. Patients do not seem to have a preference for 1 interpretation type rather than another type, although some data suggest a greater degree of patient satisfaction with telephonic interpreters or video interpreters compared with in-person interpreters.[19,23] As described later, certain clinical encounters may be best suited for a particular interpreter type.

Comparative Cost

Budgets often direct the choice of interpreter services available at a clinic or hospital. The driving assumption for this is that any cost savings for language interpretation results in a net savings to the health care system, an assumption that may be incorrect. Using ad hoc interpreters avoids an overhead expense but, as noted previously, this can cause a downstream cost because of errors in clinically important

In-person Interpreter	Video Interpreter	Telephone Interpreter
• Clinician preferred • Accurate, efficient • Considered gold standard for patient comprehension of diagnosis and treatment • Able to translate written materials	• Useful for hearing impaired individuals • Able to see body language, gestures • Readily available in many languages	• Readily available in a large number of languages • Patient privacy respected • Lower overhead cost

Fig. 1. Features of professional interpreter services.

communication. One study noted that language-discordant patients averaged higher medical costs per encounter (US$38 greater per emergency department visit and US$92 greater per inpatient stay) than patients with language-concordant physicians.[24]

Phone interpreter services are noted to be expensive on a per-minute basis (averaging two US$/min) but have the benefit of low structural overhead and only creating expense during interpretation time.[24] The service is readily available at the point of care. Video interpretation services are up to 50% more expensive than phone interpretation.[25] Video interpretation incurs more capital expense in the form of infrastructure, because of the use of tablets and mobile tablet stands. These costs can add up, and considerable infrastructure investment is needed to provide equitable distribution.

In-person interpretation has the highest cost per hour at approximately US$32 but suffers from the inefficiency of the interpreter moving locations frequently and incurring expense during inactive periods of their shifts.[24] This inefficiency leads to 60% cost savings when large health care systems move to employ telephone services as opposed to in-person interpreters.[24] Based on the logistical limitations, the in-person methodology is most cost-effective in locations with a high density of patients who are fluent in one language. As an example, many hospital systems in the United States have the population density to justify employing in-person Spanish or Arabic interpreters. Refugee resettlement sites can also employ in-person interpreters for larger populations such as the Montagnard in North Carolina or Hmong in California.[26]

PLN health ambassadors received US$25/h for their time working, independent of physicians, on increasing general community health literacy in their native languages.[16] These costs were not direct interpretation for a health encounter, so it is not easy to compare the cost-effectiveness with the other methods. This preventive investment in the community may increase healthy literacy and reduce overall health care spending. The cost-efficiency of these interventions has not been assessed but, much like wellness visits, the hypothesis is that investing in the patient's health knowledge will produce cost savings and improved health outcomes.

Underlying all of the costs outlined earlier is the difficulty with payment for these services. Medicare and most private insurers do not reimburse for interpretation services and Medicaid reimburses for these services in just 10 states throughout the United States.[27] However, the cost of failing to provide interpretation in terms of poor patient outcomes is far greater than the cost of professional interpreter services.

Special Considerations

Telehealth and telemedicine represent another potential area of health inequity for LEP individuals. Immigrant and refugee populations have considerable difficulty navigating the complex health care systems. During times of pandemics (such as that of the COVID19 [coronavirus disease 2019] pandemic) or natural disasters, this system becomes even more complicated. Multiple telemedicine platforms have partnered with interpreter services to provide audio and audiovisual capabilities for virtual visits.[28] The patient and provider satisfaction with such services is unknown at this time. As these remote services continue to expand, further research will be needed to determine the effect of these communication tools on the health outcomes of refugee and immigrant populations.

BEST PRACTICES

Working successfully with interpreters requires skill and practice (**Fig. 2**). Reviewing the patient's chart in some detail before an encounter, if possible, can help determine the best form of interpretation in the encounter.[29] The in-person interpreter has been identified by many clinicians as the preferred interpreter type. If unavailable, telephone interpreters may be preferable in encounters for patient privacy, whereas video interpreters are necessary for patients with hearing impairment. Involving the patient and family in choosing the preferred type of interpreter can facilitate a successful encounter.[30]

It can be helpful to let the interpreter know whom to expect in the examination room and any anticipated examinations or procedures. The interpreter should be treated as a collaborator and professional colleague. Interpreters can help clinicians understand

Pearls	Pitfalls
• An in-person interpreter should be seated next to the patient or slightly behind the provider	• Do not use an examination room or space too small for participants
• Communicate directly to the patient, maintaining culturally appropriate eye contact	• Do not turn to the interpreter when speaking to the patient
• Use clear, straightforward language	• Avoid special or advanced terminology
• Speak slowly and in short sequences	• Avoid interrupting the patient or interpreter
• Use the teach-back method to show comprehension	• Do not use complex sentence structure
• Encourage the interpreter to ask questions or clarifying statements	• Beware some concepts may not have an equivalent in all languages

Fig. 2. Key points for patient encounters with interpreters.

cultural norms in discussion before or after the encounter. They can also serve to describe the health care system structure to immigrants and refugees new to a large system. Allowing time to introduce the interpreter services to the patient at the start of the visit results in a more effective and efficient clinical encounter.

CLINICAL CASES

> A 21-year-old girl is brought for her initial health examination at your clinic after arrival from Nepal. Record review from her overseas medical examination reveals she had bacterial meningitis at age 1 year, resulting in hearing impairment. She has no other medical conditions per chart. The patient does not use an assistive hearing device and communicates in Nepali sign language. Her mother and father bring her to the appointment. An in-person interpreter provides interpretation services in Nepali. How would you navigate communication with this patient?

Key components of this clinical encounter include previsit planning, communicating early on with interpreters, and engaging the entire family in the visit. Before each visit with patients with LEP, the care team should discuss the strategy for effective communication and care of the patient, which should include a discussion of the plan for interpretation services. Communicating with this patient presents a unique challenge, because she communicates in Nepali sign language. Although it may seem easiest to allow parents to provide translation from Nepali to Nepali sign language and back, interpretation by family members results in a higher rate of clinically significant errors.[31] Some live interpreters are able to interpret from both Nepali and Nepali sign language into English. Alternatively, a video interpreter who can interpret from Nepali sign language to Nepali, which the live interpreter in turn interprets into English, represents another solution.

After arrival of the interpreter, introduce yourself and communicate with the interpreter regarding the individuals expected to be present in the room to facilitate a fluid clinical encounter. Allow time for the interpreters to introduce themselves to the patient. Be sure to engage the patient in her health care and elicit her concerns. Although caregiver questions and concerns should be addressed, the patient should be interviewed without her parents in the room. This approach allows clinicians to elicit the patient's full story, which she may not feel comfortable discussing in front of her parents. In addition, this will help to elicit the patient's concerns in addition to parental concerns. Professional interpreters in this setting increase patient satisfaction and improve patient outcomes.[30]

> A 29-year-old mother of two presents for care at your clinic. She is due for her Pap smear. You enter the room to find the patient, her husband, and 2 young children. The patient speaks Arabic. The patient's husband informs you that he will provide interpretation for the visit.

The founding principles of patient care include respect for the patients and their autonomy. In some clinical cases, family members may demand to provide interpretation services for the patient. Eliciting concerns from the patients and their families and allowing for discussion about the options for effective interpretation can help reduce this tension. In addition, establishing a clinical care policy to use professional interpreter services allows providers to refer to the policy and limit the use of family members as interpreters. Because many clinics use video or phone interpreters for clinical care, connecting with an Arabic interpreter while the husband is still present in the room can be helpful to establish trust. This approach can often allay fears about the skills of professional interpreters. After establishing this trust, the clinician can often ask the husband and children for privacy during the examination, thus using a culturally appropriate, professional interpreter for the visit.

Many refugees entering into the United States identify as Muslim.[32] Key principles of the Muslim faith are that of privacy and humility.[33] Many women prefer a female interpreter for sensitive interviews. Even with a female interpreter, many women prefer a telephone-only female interpreter to maximize privacy. Respecting the patient's privacy by limiting exposure, avoiding eye contact, and providing gender-concordant care when possible can further help in establishing a trusting relationship.

A 14-year-old boy presents for a routine well-child examination. You know the family well as their primary care provider for the past 5 years since arrival in the United States. His mother, who speaks French and Swahili only, joins the boy. The boy is fluent in French, Swahili, and English. He tells the nurse that he does not need an interpreter.

Providing comprehensive care to a pediatric patient must involve the entire family. Children should never be used as interpreters for parents, even in their own appointments.[34] The ACA forbids the use of children as interpreters. Using a video or telephone interpreter to elicit parental concerns allows full inclusion of the parent in the visit. The interpreter should interpret the clinician's words as well as the child's words spoken in English for the parent. It is often helpful to have the child and parent speak in a single language (in this case Swahili or French) to facilitate communication. The American Academy of Pediatrics recommends 1-on-1 time with adolescents and physicians beginning at age 11 years.[35] Describing the visit plan and importance of this independent conversation early in the visit can reduce worry and ensure comprehensive care of the adolescent. Time with the patient alone allows him to discuss concerns he may be hesitant to discuss with his mother in the room. This portion of the interview can be conducted in either English as the interpreter stands by or in his preferred language. Often, letting pediatric patients know it is clinic policy to use a professional interpreter can reduce their anxiety about translating perfectly for their parents and themselves.

CLINICS CARE POINTS

- Immigrants and refugees have higher rates of LEP and have associated poorer health outcomes.
- Professional interpreter services can improve patient outcomes and satisfaction while reducing errors.
- In-person interpretation has the highest cost but is most highly rated by clinicians. Patients variably rate this service.
- Patients may prefer telephone interpretation for privacy reasons, whereas video interpretation can be useful for hearing-impaired individuals.
- Previsit planning regarding the type of interpreter and logistics of interpretation can help to improve clinician and patient satisfaction during encounters.

ACKNOWLEDGMENTS

Specials thanks to medical librarian Laura Eynon-Way.

DISCLOSURE

The authors have nothing to disclose.

REFERENCES

1. Zong J, Batalova J. The limited English proficient population in the United States. Migration Policy Institute. 2015. Available at: https://www.migrationpolicy.org/article/limited-english-proficient-population-united-states. Accessed April 19, 2020.
2. An increasingly diverse linguistic profile: corrected data from the 2016 census. The Daily. 2017. Available at: https://www150.statcan.gc.ca/n1/daily-quotidien/170817/dq170817a-eng.htm. Accessed April 19, 2020.
3. National Council on Interpreting in Health Care: FAQs-healthcare professionals. Available at: https://www.ncihc.org/faqs-for-healthcare-professionals. Accessed April 19, 2020.
4. Berdahl TA, Kirby JB. Patient-provider communication disparities by limited English proficiency (LEP): trends from the US Medical Expenditure Panel Survey, 2006–2015. J Gen Intern Med 2019;34(8):1434–40.
5. Griswold KS, Pottie K, Kim I, et al. Strengthening effective preventive services for refugee populations: toward communities of solution. Public Health Rev 2018; 39:3.
6. Jang Y, Yoon H, Park NS, et al. Health vulnerability of immigrants with limited English proficiency: a study of older Korean Americans. J Am Geriatr Soc 2016; 64(7):1498–502.
7. Improving patient safety systems for limited-English-proficient (LEP) patients: a guide for hospitals. Agency for Health Research and Quality. 2012. Available at: https://www.ahrq.gov/teamstepps/lep/hospitalguide/lephospitalguide.html#sl19. Accessed April 19, 2020.
8. Title VI of the Civil Rights Act of 1964: Policy guidance on the prohibition against national origin discrimination as it affects persons with limited English proficiency. Federal Register. 2019. Available at: https://www.federalregister.gov/documents/2000/08/30/00-22140/title-vi-of-the-civil-rights-act-of-1964-policy-guidance-on-the-prohibition-against-national-origin. Accessed May 15, 2020.
9. Nondiscrimination in health programs and activities. Federal Register. 2016. Available at: https://www.federalregister.gov/documents/2016/05/18/2016-11458/nondiscrimination-in-health-programs-and-activities#h-48. Accessed April 30, 2020.
10. Bowen S. Language barriers in access to health care 2001. 2001. Available at: https://www.canada.ca/en/health-canada/services/health-care-system/reports-publications/health-care-accessibility/language-barriers.html. Accessed April 19, 2020.
11. The National Council on Interpreting in Health Care, working papers series: a national code of ethics for interpreters in healthcare, 2004. Available at: http://www.ncihc.org. Accessed April 19, 2020.
12. CLAS Standards – think cultural health. Available at: https://thinkculturalhealth.hhs.gov/clas/standards. Accessed April 19, 2020.

13. The blueprint for advancing and sustaining CLAS policy and practice. 2013. https://thinkculturalhealth.hhs.gov/clas/blueprint. Accessed May 15, 2020.
14. Passel J, Cohn D. Pew Research Center. U.S. unauthorized immigrants are more proficient in English, more educated than a decade ago. 2019. Available at: https://www.pewresearch.org/fact-tank/2019/05/23/u-s-undocumented-immigrants-are-more-proficient-in-english-more-educated-than-a-decade-ago. Accessed July 11, 2020.
15. Capps R, Newland K, Fratze S, et al. The integration outcomes of US refugees: successes and challenges. Washington, DC: Migration Policy Institute; 2015.
16. Johnson RM, Shepard L, Van Den Berg R, et al. A novel approach to improve health literacy in immigrant communities. Health Lit Res Pract 2019;3(3 Suppl): S15–24.
17. Schwei RJ, Schroeder M, Ejebe I, et al. Limited English proficient patients' perceptions of when interpreters are needed and how the decision to utilize interpreters is made. Health Commun 2018;33(12):1503–8.
18. Cheng EM, Chen A, Cunningham W. Primary language and receipt of recommended health care among Hispanics in the United States. J Gen Intern Med 2007; 22(Suppl 2):283–8.
19. Crossman KL, Wiener E, Roosevelt G, et al. Interpreters: telephonic, in-person interpretation and bilingual providers. Pediatrics 2010;125(3):e631–8.
20. Lion KC, Brown JC, Ebel BE, et al. Effect of telephone vs video interpretation on parent comprehension, communication, and utilization in the Pediatric Emergency Department: a randomized clinical trial. JAMA Pediatr 2015;169(12): 1117–25.
21. Flores G, Abreu M, Barone CP, et al. Errors of medical interpretation and their potential clinical consequences: a comparison of professional versus ad hoc versus no interpreters. Ann Emerg Med 2012;60(5):545–53.
22. Karliner LS, Jacobs EA, Chen AH, et al. Do professional interpreters improve clinical care for patients with limited English proficiency? A systematic review of the literature. Health Serv Res 2007;42(2):727–54.
23. Locatis C, Williamson D, Gould-Kabler C, et al. Comparing in-person, video, and telephonic medical interpretation. J Gen Intern Med 2010;25:345–50.
24. Masland MC, Lou C, Snowden L. Use of communication technologies to cost-effectively increase the availability of interpretation services in healthcare settings. Telemed J E Health 2010;16(6):739–45.
25. Jacobs B, Ryan AM, Henrichs KS, et al. Medical Interpreters in Outpatient Practice. Ann Fam Med 2018;16(1):70–6.
26. Green AR, Nze C. Language-based inequity in health care: who is the "poor historian"? AMA J Ethics 2017;19(3):263–71.
27. Ku L, Flores G. Pay now or pay later: providing interpreter services in health care. Health Aff 2005;24(2).
28. Schultz TR, Richards M, Gasko H, et al. Telehealth: experience of first 120 consultations delivered from a new refugee telehealth clinic. Intern Med J 2014;44: 981–5.
29. Hadziabdic E, Hjelm K. Working with interpreters: practical advice for use of an interpreter in healthcare. Int J Evid Based Healthc 2013;11(1):69–76.
30. Juckett G, Unger K. Appropriate use of medical interpreters. Am Fam Physician 2014;90(7):476–80.
31. Flores G, Laws B, May S, et al. Errors in medical interpretation and their potential clinical consequences in pediatric encounters. Pediatrics 2003;111(1):6–14.
32. Connor P, Krogstad JM. The number of refugees admitted to the US has fallen, especially among Muslims. Pew Research Center. 2018. Available at: https://

Achieving access to primary care can be difficult for immigrant and refugee populations. Immigrants use primary care less, in a way that suggests inequitable access rather than less need.[4,5] Immigrants also have less access to preventive care than native-born populations,[6] likely because of a variety of factors (eg, insurance status, language barriers). Even when immigrant patients do have access to services, observers have noted a mismatch between what immigrant patients want from health care and what is provided in the US system, possibly contributing to underuse of health care and subsequent health disparities.[7] Similar barriers to care are thought to be present for refugee populations as well, although nationally representative data have been noted to be sparse.[2]

This mismatch can be harmful to both immigrant and refugee patients' experiences of health care and providers' ability to take care of these patients. A systematic review of the literature suggested that immigrant patients are less satisfied with health care and experience more discrimination.[4] On the provider side, physicians' overestimation of alignment with their patients' beliefs about health is exacerbated when patients are of a different race than the physician or are black or Hispanic.[8] This overestimation may contribute to provider dissatisfaction with patients' efforts to manage their health conditions: providers have been found to be less satisfied when taking care of immigrant patients, with the main source of dissatisfaction being providers' impressions of their immigrant patients as lacking understanding of prevention and management of chronic disease.[9]

The solutions required to provide quality cross-cultural care are not simple or straightforward, but improving providers' ability to understand their patients has been articulated as a key step.[10] To begin to understand their cross-cultural patients, providers must be able to conceptualize how culture may affect all parts of the health care system. In 1978, Kleinman[11] advanced the concept of "medicine as a cultural system," and, with colleagues, advanced the case for incorporating cross-cultural perspectives and anthropologic research ("clinical social science") into health care education. In their words, "the incorporation of clinical social science is essential if physicians are to understand, respond to, and help patients deal with the concerns they bring to the doctor."[11,12] To assist in this task, this article discusses the different ways culture affects health care, in terms of patient-related factors, health care provider–related factors, and health care system–related factors. This article also describes some interventions and best practices that draw on the incorporation of culture into health care and that thus may be effective for building the crucial cross-cultural understanding between providers and their immigrant and refugee patients.

CULTURAL FACTORS AFFECTING PRIMARY CARE
Patient Factors

How patients conceptualize their illnesses
How patients conceptualize their health and the factors that affect their health can vary across cultures and can be a key contributor to a lack of understanding between provider and patient. This conceptualization is often referred to as an explanatory model, which can include explanations about cause of illness, onset of symptoms, pathophysiology, course of illness, and treatment.[11] Eliciting an immigrant patient's explanatory model for a given illness is a key task for a provider seeking a better understanding of a patient, because conflicts between a patient's explanatory model and the provider's model can drive problems in patient care.[11]

To demonstrate the concept of the explanatory model, Armstrong and Swartzman[7] described 3 different models that are common in different cultures. First, they outline the biomedical model (dominant in Western cultures), which is characterized by the view that illness is understood to occur through biochemical processes and that interventions involve a biological or chemical correction. Next, they discuss the traditional Chinese medical model, where health is determined by the balance (or imbalance) of certain elements, including both biological and social elements, and where interventions, therefore, are designed to restore balance to the individual. In addition, they describe the Ayurvedic medicine tradition, commonly found in South Asian cultures, in which balance between 3 specific elements found in nature determines health, and these elements can be affected by factors such as emotion, the weather, and food.

Several commentators have proposed general frameworks for patients' explanatory models and ways to incorporate cultural differences into these frameworks. Angel and Williams[13] proposed that individuals and cultures differ in beliefs about health on 2 dimensions: the degree to which illness is privately observable (subjective) versus being publicly observable (objective), and the degree to which illness occurs in the body versus in the mind. In their systemic review, Hughner and Kleine[14] identified 18 different lay beliefs about health, such as that health is equilibrium, health is freedom, and health is genetics, although they did not focus on how different cultures emphasized these different themes. Kleinman and colleagues[12] made a distinction between the concepts of disease and illness, arguing that disease is defined by malfunctioning biological or physiologic processes, whereas illness is defined by the person's reaction to disease, which may be shaped by personal, interpersonal, and cultural factors. They observed that health care professionals overemphasize concepts of disease, whereas lay patients overemphasize concepts of illness, and posit that both disease and illness are explanatory models that need to be accounted for when addressing health. Culture-bound syndromes, which are culture-specific aberrant experiences that have not been well accounted for by existing psychiatric disorder classification systems, can be thought of as specific examples of explanatory models. The most recent fifth revision to the Diagnostic and Statistical Manual of Mental Disorders (DSM-5) evolved from describing these experiences as "culture-bound" to "cultural concepts of distress," which reflects a broader view that all mental distress is culturally framed.[15]

How patients conceptualize their care

Culture can also influence how patients think about the care they receive, including their view of the provider-patient relationship as well as their view of what treatments they prefer. Along with their distinction between the biomedically focused disease and experientially focused illness explanatory models, Kleinman and colleagues[12] described different views of treatment, comparing curing, which addresses disease by resolving the maladaptive biological process, with healing, which addresses illness by providing a meaningful explanation and attending to the personal, interpersonal, and community issues affected by illness. Different cultures emphasize these 2 views to varying degrees, which can set patients' expectations about the roles their health care providers play and about the treatments that may be offered.

Cultural effects on treatment preferences can be observed in a variety of treatment contexts, such as end-of-life care, asthma, depression, colds, insomnia, and back pain.[16–20] Immigrants to the United States bring health practices with them, which they sometimes prefer to the prevalent Western health practices or wish to use in combination.[19] Goals for treatment are also subject to cultural effects; for example, patients from individualistic cultures may value self-focused symptom relief most highly, whereas patients from collectivistic cultures may place a higher value on regaining their ability to fulfill community roles.[7] Gaps between patients and health care providers in understanding beliefs about treatment may lead to non-adherence to treatment recommendations, patient's distrust in the provider-patient relationship, provider dissatisfaction, and overall missed opportunities to address health problems effectively.

Provider Factors

Cultural humility versus cultural competence

Culture also influences how health care providers approach caring for their patients, often in ways that are consequential for immigrant health. In an effort to address health care disparities, health care systems identified so-called cultural competence as a key goal, despite some challenges in developing a consistent definition.[21] At the level of the health care providers, cultural competence can be defined as the "knowledge, tools, and skills to better understand and manage sociocultural issues in the clinical encounter."[21] In addition, some definitions of cultural competence also emphasize the role of increasing providers' self-awareness of their own cultural backgrounds and their perspectives about other cultures.[22] These views of cultural competence imply a goal of providers' attaining proficiency with regard to how cultural differences may present in the clinic.

The concept of cultural competence, or perhaps the way in which cultural competence has been defined, has attracted numerous criticisms, including a lack of self-awareness about ethnocentrism in health care, an oversimplification of culture as being equivalent to racial/ethnic group identity, a view of cultural competence as a task with an end point rather than an ongoing process, and a lack of agenda for addressing inequalities.[23] Tervalon and Murray-Garcia[24] proposed "cultural humility" as an alternative concept, which differs from common cultural competence frameworks by its emphasis on ongoing commitment to self-evaluation around working with cultural differences; acknowledgment of, and efforts to challenge, power imbalances in provider-patient relationships; and developing partnerships with patients' communities. As a concept, cultural humility carries additional complexity compared with the proficiency-focused and skill-focused cultural competence but does offer a tighter link to structural inequalities that affect immigrant and refugee patients.

Systems factors

Patients and providers face structural barriers to providing care that is culturally informed. Given the demographics of the health care workforce, immigrant and refugee patients are likely to see providers of different racial/ethnic backgrounds than themselves, which can result in less patient involvement in care.[25] Some health care organizations lack basic infrastructure for providing culturally informed care, such as lack of linguistically and culturally appropriate educational materials or health promotion programs, or even appropriate signage.[25] When organizations have tried to implement strategies to address gaps in culturally informed care, a lack of precision in defining cultural competence has led to resistance and a lack of successful implementation.[26]

Interventions/practice tools

Examples are presented next of interventions intended to strengthen culturally appropriate health care at 3 different levels: the patient encounter, provider training, and broader systems.

Explanatory model interview
At the patient encounter level, a useful strategy for incorporating cultural considerations into the care of immigrant and refugee patients is to elicit the patient's explanatory model. When describing explanatory models and their relevance to clinical
practice, Kleinman and colleagues[12] suggested a series of questions that can serve
as a patient-centered interview that assesses patients' beliefs about their illness, their
expectations for treatment, and their treatment goals. Lloyd and colleagues[27] built on
this work by developing a 30-minute to 45-minute semistructured clinical interview
that probes the nature of the problem, help-seeking efforts, expectations for the interaction with the health care provider, and beliefs related to health. They found that this
interview was able to capture variability in explanatory models across cultures, based
on the results in the different populations they tested with the interview questions.
Mauksch and Roesler[28] advanced a strategy for collecting additional contextual details in the explanatory model interview by asking circular questions, which are questions asked about a person or persons in a relationship with the patient (eg, family
members, peers). For example, they suggest asking questions such as, "Do others
in your family think this is a serious or benign illness?" This approach positions the
clinician to gain an understanding of the family system's effects on the patient's
explanatory model, which could be particularly valuable for patients with collectivistic
cultural backgrounds. Regardless of the specific questions asked, eliciting the explanatory model is an important step for clinicians forming an understanding of how culture
might be playing a role in a patient's health.

After eliciting the explanatory model for a patient, it is crucial for health care providers to then incorporate this newly formed understanding into the treatment plan.
Kleinman and colleagues[12] provided the important insight that health care providers
have their own explanatory model of the illness, and, as such, the patient's and provider's models must be compared transparently in the interaction, with ample opportunity given for open communication around the differences between these models.
They recommended that this comparison of explanatory models be followed up
with negotiation of a treatment plan that accounts for both models; they note that
this negotiation might not require discrepant explanatory models to be changed,
because the treatment plan might be able to accommodate the various explanatory
models. Carrillo and colleagues[29] outlined specific strategies for negotiating explanatory models and treatment, which emphasize the role of open discussion around differences in explanatory models and treatment priorities, as well as the importance of
shared decision making about the treatment plan. For example, a patient with hypertension may present with an explanatory model that this problem is episodic and
linked to discrete stressful events requiring as-needed treatment, compared with
the provider's model of hypertension as an ongoing condition requiring regular medication. Negotiating around treatment may involve both openly discussing the
discrepant explanatory models and agreeing to a treatment plan that can accommodate both explanatory models, such as the patient using herbal tea as needed after a
stressful event, and also taking medication daily to address the ongoing aspect of the
condition.

Building cultural humility at the clinician level
Strategies for improving culturally informed care through provider education have also
been studied. Carrillo and colleagues[29] developed an 8-hour curriculum for residents
and medical students that starts at building a foundational understanding of culture
and explanatory models and takes trainees through modules designed to increase
their ability to elicit explanatory models and engage in the cultural negotiation

described earlier. Chang and colleagues[30] constructed a model curriculum for cultural humility based on contemporary Chinese immigrants' experiences that has 4 elements:

1. Self-questioning and self-critique around what a person's assumptions about the world are and how they are developed
2. Immersion, which takes the form of taking perspectives around patients' experiences
3. Active listening
4. Negotiation

Fisher-Borne and colleagues[23] advocate a self-assessment and organizational assessment of cultural humility along 2 dimensions: critical self-reflection (eg, "How do my cultural identities shape my worldview?," "How is culture defined organizationally?") and addressing power imbalances (eg, "What social and economic barriers affect a client's ability to receive effective care?," "What are the organizational structures that encourage action to address inequalities?"). They suggest that this self-assessment can then lead to the development of curricula and teaching activities to address the specific areas for growth revealed through assessment.

Culturally specific services/shifts to the structure of health care

Some organizations seeking to build a better understanding of culture and health have implemented system-level interventions. For example, Dominicé Dao and colleagues[31] addressed the challenge of maintaining uptake of explanatory model interviewing by developing a hospital-wide cultural consultation service to support clinicians who have difficulties with cross-cultural care. In this service, consultants conduct an explanatory model–style interview, ideally with the referring provider present, resulting in a consultation report for the care team to draw on for guidance and feedback given directly to the referring provider. The investigators reported that the referring clinicians endorsed high satisfaction with this service, because of the information gained about the patient context as well as the opportunity to observe how the consultant conducted the interview.

Anderson and colleagues[32] describe 5 types of system-level interventions that might contribute to cultural understanding in health care:

1. Programs to recruit and retain staff representative of the communities they serve
2. Language access services
3. Cultural competence training for providers
4. Linguistically and culturally appropriate health education materials
5. Integrating health care services into culturally specific settings

In a review of these types of system-level interventions, Truong and colleagues[33] found evidence of positive effects on access to and use of services, but only weak evidence for positive effects on patient-level outcomes; they noted methodological issues in the studies they reviewed related to a lack of objective measures and well-validated measures for outcomes.

SUMMARY

Culture's influence on health can be observed at a variety of levels for immigrant patients: how the patients think about their health and medical treatments; whether providers are able to use cultural humility in order to build an understanding of how the patients' cultural differences might affect their care; and how accommodating (or hostile) health care systems are to patients from diverse cultural backgrounds. Although challenges exist at each of these levels, researchers have identified promising strategies to address these challenges in the patient encounter, in provider training, and in the types of services health care systems provide. However, for primary care clinicians (or practices) attempting to provide culturally informed care to immigrant and refugee populations, it is important to recognize that there is no one-size-fits-all strategy or playbook for achieving culturally informed care. Depending on the cultural backgrounds and specific health needs of the populations being served, as well as the cultural backgrounds of providers and staff, consistent with the concept of cultural humility, there is much room for self-reflection, self-critique, and attempts to address inequalities, especially in the context of a lifelong process of improvement.

CLINICS CARE POINTS

- When discussing a health condition, elicit the patient's explanatory model using Kleinman and colleagues'[12] questions and circular questioning and share your own explanatory model.
- Negotiate the treatment plan with these explanatory models in mind; seek to find a treatment plan that can accommodate discrepant explanatory models.
- Consider developing a cultural consultation service, or develop informal avenues for cultural consultations, for clinicians to assist each other with eliciting patients' explanatory models and incorporating them into treatment.

DISCLOSURE

The authors have nothing to disclose.

REFERENCES

1. Choi SH. Testing healthy immigrant effects among late life immigrants in the united states: using multiple indicators. J Aging Health 2012;24(3):475–506.
2. Reed HE, Barbosa GY. Investigating the refugee health disadvantage among the U.S. immigrant population. J Immigr Refug Stud 2017;15(1):53–70.
3. Calvo R, Hawkins SS. Disparities in quality of healthcare of children from immigrant families in the US. Matern Child Health J 2015;19(10):2223–32.
4. Pitkin Derose K, Bahney BW, Lurie N, et al. Review: immigrants and health care access, quality, and cost. Med Care Res Rev 2009;66(4):355–408.
5. Uiters E, Devillé W, Foets M, et al. Differences between immigrant and non-immigrant groups in the use of primary medical care; a systematic review. BMC Health Serv Res 2009;9(1):76.
6. Singh GK, Rodriguez-Lainz A, Kogan MD. Immigrant health inequalities in the united states: use of eight major national data systems. ScientificWorldJournal 2013;2013:1–21.
7. Armstrong TL, Swartzman LC. Cross-cultural differences in illness models and expectations for the health care provider-client/patient interaction. In: handbook of Cultural Health Psychology. Elsevier; 2001. p. 63–84. https://doi.org/10.1016/B978-012402771-8/50005-2.
8. Street RL, Haidet P. How well do doctors know their patients? Factors affecting physician understanding of patients' health beliefs. J Gen Intern Med 2011; 26(1):21–7.

9. Kamath CC, O'Fallon WM, Offord KP, et al. Provider satisfaction in clinical encounters with ethnic immigrant patients. Mayo Clin Proc 2003;78:1353–60. Elsevier.

10. Betancourt J, Green A, Carillo JE. The challenges of cross-cultural healthcare-diversity, ethics, and the medical encounter. Bioethics Forum 2000;16:27–32. MIDWEST BIOETHICS CENTER.

11. Kleinman A. Concepts and a model for the comparison of medical systems as cultural systems. Soc Sci Med 1978;12:85–93.

12. Kleinman A, Eisenberg L, Good B. Culture, illness, and care: clinical lessons from anthropologic and cross-cultural research. Ann Intern Med 1978;88(2):251–8.

13. Angel RJ, Williams K. Cultural models of health and illness. In: handbook of multicultural mental health. Elsevier; 2000. p. 25–44.

14. Hughner RS, Kleine SS. Views of health in the lay sector: a compilation and review of how individuals think about health. Health (London) 2004;8(4):395–422.

15. Ventriglio A, Ayonrinde O, Bhugra D. Relevance of culture-bound syndromes in the 21st century: culture-bound syndromes in 21st century. Psychiatry Clin Neurosci 2016;70(1):3–6.

16. Cherniack EP, Ceron-Fuentes J, Florez H, et al. Influence of race and ethnicity on alternative medicine as a self-treatment preference for common medical conditions in a population of multi-ethnic urban elderly. Complement Ther Clin Pract 2008;14(2):116–23.

17. Jimenez DE, Bartels SJ, Cardenas V, et al. Cultural beliefs and mental health treatment preferences of ethnically diverse older adult consumers in primary care. Am J Geriatr Psychiatry 2012;20(6):533–42.

18. Lang AJ. Mental health treatment preferences of primary care patients. J Behav Med 2005;28(6):581–6.

19. Shaw SJ, Huebner C, Armin J, et al. The role of culture in health literacy and chronic disease screening and management. J Immigr Minor Health 2009; 11(6):460–7.

20. Thomas R, Wilson DM, Justice C, et al. A literature review of preferences for end-of-life care in developed countries by individuals with different cultural affiliations and ethnicity. J Hosp Palliat Nurs 2008;10(3):142–61.

21. Betancourt JR, Green AR, Carrillo JE, et al. Defining cultural competence: a practical framework for addressing racial/ethnic disparities in health and health care. Public Health Rep 2003;118:10.

22. Kutob RM, Bormanis J, Crago M, et al. Cultural competence education for practicing physicians: lessons in cultural humility, nonjudgmental behaviors, and health beliefs elicitation. J Contin Educ Health Prof 2013;33(3):164–73.

23. Fisher-Borne M, Cain JM, Martin SL. From mastery to accountability: cultural humility as an alternative to cultural competence. Soc Work Educ 2015;34(2): 165–81.

24. Tervalon M, Murray-García J. Cultural humility versus cultural competence: a critical distinction in defining physician training outcomes in multicultural education. J Health Care Poor Underserved 1998;9(2):117–25.

25. Castillo RJ, Guo KL. A framework for cultural competence in health care organizations. Health Care Manag 2011;30(3):205–14.

26. Engebretson J, Mahoney J, Carlson ED. Cultural competence in the era of evidence-based practice. J Prof Nurs 2008;24(3):172–8.

27. Lloyd KR, Jacob KS, Patel V, et al. The development of the Short Explanatory Model Interview (SEMI) and its use among primary-care attenders with common mental disorders. Psychol Med 1998;28(5):1231–7.

28. Mauksch LB, Roesler T. Expanding the context of the patient's explanatory model using circular questioning. Fam Syst Med 1990;8(1):3–13.
29. Carrillo JE, Green AR, Betancourt JR. Cross-cultural primary care: a patient-based approach. Ann Intern Med 1999;130(10):829.
30. Chang E, Simon M, Dong X. Integrating cultural humility into health care professional education and training. Adv Health Sci Educ Theory Pract 2012;17(2): 269–78.
31. Dominicé Dao M, Inglin S, Vilpert S, et al. The relevance of clinical ethnography: reflections on 10 years of a cultural consultation service. BMC Health Serv Res 2018;18(1):19.
32. Anderson LM, Scrimshaw SC, Fullilove MT, et al. Culturally competent healthcare systems. Am J Prev Med 2003;24(3):68–79.
33. Truong M, Paradies Y, Priest N. Interventions to improve cultural competency in healthcare: a systematic review of reviews. BMC Health Serv Res 2014; 14(1):99.

Common Infectious Diseases

Kevin Pottie, MD, CCFP, MClSc, FCFP[a],*, Vincent Girard, BHSc[b]

KEYWORDS

- Refugees • Immigrants • Infectious diseases • Tuberculosis • HIV • Hepatitis B
- Hepatitis C • Intestinal parasites

KEY POINTS

- Immigrants and refugees benefit from evidence-based global health screening for specific infectious diseases.
- Common diseases that may accompany an immigrant or refugee migrating from tropical countries include tuberculosis, human immunodeficiency virus, hepatitis, and intestinal parasites.
- Other infectious diseases that may warrant treatment when present include malaria, chikungunya, Chagas, scabies, and COVID-19.

INTRODUCTION

Front-line clinicians and public health officials often provide health care to immigrants, refugees, and other migrants from a wide range of countries, languages, and socio-economic backgrounds.[1] Many clinicians may not know where to focus their patient-centered approach, which patient concerns to address, and which infectious diseases may benefit from screening and treatment. Research suggests that fear of clinical uncertainty, medical legal concerns, and language differences are all potent clinician deterrents to providing timely immigrant and refugee services.[2,3] Developing an interest and positive regard toward newcomers and their families; openness to different languages, cultures, and religions; focusing on the presenting patient complaint; working in interdisciplinary teams; and then allowing clinical guidelines to improve the scope of screening can turn a chore into an intellectually and culturally enriching work environment.[2,3]

Clinical guidelines frame the benefits and harms of interventions and summarize cost, values, and health equity for practitioners and their refugee patients.[3–6] Indeed, infectious disease guidelines recommend that primary health care and public health practitioners address detectable and preventable illness for newly arriving immigrants

[a] Department of Family Medicine, School of Epidemiology Public Health and Preventive Medicine, University of Ottawa, Ottawa, Ontario, Canada; [b] University of Ottawa, 600 Peter Morand Crescent #201, Ottawa, ON K1G 5Z3, Canada
* Corresponding author. Bruyere Family Medicine Centre, 75 Bruyere Street, Ottawa K1N 5C8, Canada.
E-mail address: kpottie@uottawa.ca
Twitter: @kevinpottie (K.P.)

Prim Care Clin Office Pract 48 (2021) 45–55
https://doi.org/10.1016/j.pop.2020.11.002
0095-4543/21/© 2020 Elsevier Inc. All rights reserved.

and refugees; for example, there are clinical guidelines in Canada,[1,7] the United States (Centers for Disease Control and Prevention [CDC]),[8] Australia,[9] and countries in the European Union/European Economic Area.[10] These clinical and public health guidelines are now supporting clinicians and the development of a global refugee and migrant health network.[11]

EVIDENCE-BASED GUIDELINE DEVELOPMENT

Evidence-based medicine (EBM) represents the integration of clinical expertise, patients' values, and best available evidence in the process of decision-making related to patient health care (**Fig. 1**).[4,5] Clinical guidelines can improve uptake and health outcomes related to health services, even more so when they are tailored for specific populations.[1–3] GRADE methods use evidence in a structured and transparent way to inform decisions in the context of clinical recommendations, coverage decisions, and health system or public health recommendations and decisions.[6] **Fig. 1** illustrates the constellation of experts involved in the production of evidence-based guidelines. Immigrant and refugee populations are underrepresented in randomized controlled trials and other intervention research. When migrant-specific studies are lacking, indirect evidence (ie, studies on general populations that can be extrapolated to interventions that are targeted toward migrants) are used. The GRADE approach states that indirect population or intervention evidence is justified, but this evidence must be downgraded a level of certainty where serious indirectness concerns exist.[12]

Indeed, guidelines help us develop clinical networks and focus on our research. In the 1990s, tropical medicine guidelines from the field were directly converted to refugee health guidelines. Rare and often difficult-to-treat diseases became screening standards for refugee medicine. However, after refugees leave the endemic countries

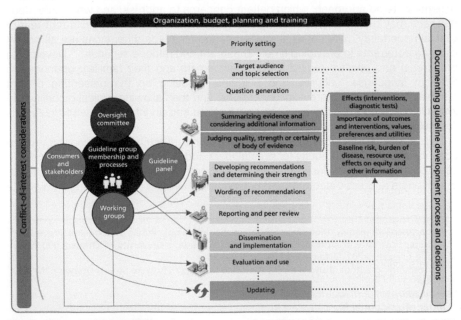

Fig. 1. Diagram of the guideline development process. (*From* Schünemann HJ, Wiercioch W, Etxeandia I, et al. Guidelines 2.0: systematic development of a comprehensive checklist for a successful guideline enterprise. CMAJ. 2014;186(3):E128; with permission.)

they rarely have trouble with such diseases and most often these diseases resolve without any diagnosis or treatment. Tropical disease scares led to overscreening, overtreatment, and clinician anxiety.[1] The next decade saw the development of evidence-based refugee health guidelines. These guidelines eliminated the routine testing of rare tropical diseases but focused on certain problematic infectious diseases. These guidelines identified evidence and gaps in evidence and have played a key role in the professionalization of immigrant and refugee health care. Priority diseases guidelines now focus on burden, effectiveness of treatment, and delivery feasibility and equity (fairness).[11] The CDC provides guidance for screening and prevention of infectious disease among newly arrived refugees to the United States (**Box 1**).

COVID-19 AND REFUGEES

COVID-19 has emerged as a humbling and insidious pandemic. As in the early days of human immunodeficiency virus (HIV), we have struggled to understand modes of transmission and we have only gradually come to recognize that migration status, living conditions, and socioeconomic status all play an important role in transmission and mortality. COVID-19 reports suggest living arrangements, packed commuter vans, and close proximity while working with meat processing contributed to the outbreaks in temporary migrant workers in Canada; more research is pending.[13] Refugee patients are at risk when they must accept poor living arrangements and must continue to work in high-risk fields such as long-term care or other front-line professions.[14] In addition, they may not understand the latest evidence and recommendations due to lack of information being provided in their native languages. Evidence from the United States has shown that ethnoracial status leads to higher mortality.[15] See the Micah Brickhill-Atkinson and Fern R. Hauck's article, "Impact of COVID-19 on Resettled Refugees," in this issue for more details about the effects of COVID-19 on refugees, immigrants, and asylum seekers.

This article focuses on infectious diseases that have emerged as priority for refugee populations and thus for clinicians who care for refugee patients, specifically tuberculosis (TB), human immunodeficiency virus (HIV), hepatitis B and C, vaccine preventable diseases, and intestinal parasites.

PRIORITY INFECTIOUS DISEASE FOR REFUGEES
Tuberculosis

TB remains a major preventable and treatable infectious disease in refugee populations.[1] Most of the transmission occurs via respiratory droplets that cause pulmonary infection. Poor nutrition, difficult living arrangements, and prison and hospital confinement all contribute to cause this infection.[1] The United States, Canada, Australia, and New Zealand have integrated chest radiograph screening within their migration programs. Programs that identify active TB will immediately treat TB. Latent TB refers to an infection with inactive TB bacteria; most (>90%) of these inactive bacteria will not reactivate in patients with good nutrition, negative HIV status, and who have adequate living conditions.[16] Many health systems in the United States and other countries will require testing to detect possible latent TB or unrecognized active TB. The classic treatment of latent TB includes daily isoniazid for 6 or 9 months. Three months of once weekly isoniazid and rifapentine is currently the preferred treatment in the United States.[17] Daily rifampin for 4 months or daily isoniazid plus rifampin for 3 months are alternatives. Additional information regarding screening is described in the Kelly Reese and Brianna Moyer's article, "Refugee Medical Screening"; and Shruti

Box 1
Summary of Centers for Disease Control and Prevention clinical guidance statements for screening and vaccination for infectious diseases among newly arrived migrants

Tuberculosis
  In the United States, most refugees undergo overseas screening for TB through a history, physical examination, and chest radiograph. Those with known HIV infection must provide sputum for microscopy and culture for *Mycobacterium tuberculosis.* As such domestic screening is rarely necessary. Interferon gamma release assay and tuberculin skin test should be used for domestic screening.

HIV
  Screening should be offered to all refugees; opt-out screening may also be considered due to the significant benefit of highly active antiretroviral therapy. If HIV positive, link to care and treatment as per clinical guidelines. Conventional antibody testing, rapid diagnostic tests, and nucleic acid tests are the commonly used testing modalities.
Hepatitis B
  Offer screening for hepatitis B (HBsAg, HBcAb, and HBsAb) to migrants born in intermediate (2%–7%) or high (≥8%) prevalence countries including infants and children.

Schistosomiasis
  Presumptive treatment is offered for most refugees from sub-Saharan Africa overseas unless medically contraindicated. If not treated overseas, this population should be presumptively treated on arrival. If a contraindication to praziquantel exists, a test and treat approach is appropriate. Testing through serology, stool and urine testing for eggs, and urine analysis for red blood cells.
Strongyloidiasis
  Overseas presumptive treatment with ivermectin for most refugee populations unless contraindicated. On arrival, either presumptive treatment or test and treat approach. Testing through *Strongyloides* IgG testing and stool ova and parasite testing.
Vaccine-preventable diseases
  Only documented vaccines should count toward the immunization record; verbal accounts are insufficient. In some cases, revaccination may be indicated if the validity of documentation is in question or severe pediatric malnutrition at the time of administration.

  HIV screening is strongly recommended as part of the domestic examination, as certain live-virus vaccines (such as MMR and varicella) are to be avoided in those with moderate to severe immunosuppression.

  Vaccinations should be given according to the host country immunization schedule. Combination vaccines can be used, and if the patient is unwilling to receive a large number of injections at once, prioritization in order of administration should be done by the clinician.

HBV vaccination among individuals who are nonimmune by serologic testing.

Varicella and HAV serology may be performed before immunization.

Children given the oral polio vaccine in or after April 2016 should be revaccinated with the inactivated polio vaccine.

Hepatitis C
Offer hepatitis C screening to detect HCV antibodies in ≥18-year-old migrants from HCV-endemic countries (≥2%) and all those born between 1945 and 1965 or having certain risk factors (such as HIV infection, injection drug use, and receipt of organs and certain blood products). Screening tests are done through anti-HCV, recombinant immunoblot assay (RIBA), and HCV RNA polymerase chain reaction (PCR).

Abbreviations: HAV, hepatitis A virus; HBcAb, hepatitis B core antibody; HBsAb, hepatitis B surface antibody; HBsAg, hepatitis B surface antigen; HBV, hepatitis B virus; HCV, hepatitis C virus; IgG; immunoglobulin G.

Data from Centers for Disease Control and Prevention. Guidelines for the U.S. domestic medical examination for newly arriving refugees. Available at: https://www.cdc.gov/immigrantrefugeehealth/guidelines/domestic/domestic-guidelines.html Accessed July 28, 2019.

Simha and Amy C. Brown's article, "Preventive Care in Children and Adolescents," in this issue.

Human Immunideficiency Virus

In Africa in the 1970s, HIV was called Slim disease, as most patients became severally cachectic and were often coinfected with TB (**Fig. 2**). Our knowledge about HIV transmission has become a useful science, with shared intravenous drugs, anal intercourse, and several other sexual practices placing individuals at risk. HIV-related stigma has played a large role in delaying diagnosis and treatment.[18] Community-based HIV rapid testing has become an evidence-based standard in Africa and parts of the United States.[19] Canada has integrated HIV testing into its migration program to support early treatment on resettlement. In vulnerable communities consider saliva-based or finger-prick rapid HIV testing. In resource-rich locations, guidelines recommend serologic testing for both HIV p24 antigen and HIV antibody to reduce the risk of missing early (eclipse period) infection. A positive result should be promptly followed with confirmatory testing. Treatment has gone from 34 pills a day in 1996 to one combination pill a day, and costs are no longer a barrier for most resettled refugees, but in the context of HIV-related stigma, a community-based test site and team can improve the uptake of testing, and the uptake of counseling for treatment and prevention. Community-based primary care may now provide treatment; however, specialized HIV clinics continue to play an expert role in care.

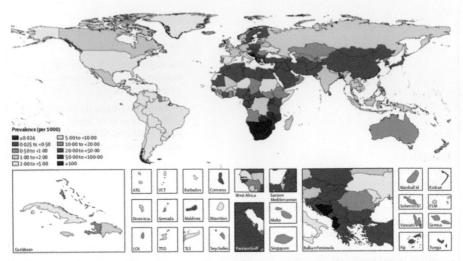

Fig. 2. Countries most affected by HIV. (*From* GBD 2017 HIV collaborators. Global, regional, and national incidence, prevalence, and mortality of HIV, 1980-2017, and forecasts to 2030, for 195 countries and territories: a systematic analysis for the Global Burden of Diseases, Injuries, and Risk Factors Study 2017. Lancet HIV. 2019;6(12):e847.)

Hepatitis

Hepatitis has emerged in the twenty-first century as a silent killer, due to chronic hepatitis and hepatocellular carcinoma. Many populations in Asia, the Middle East, and Africa are at high risk for hepatitis exposure, and thus refugee clinicians should screen the resettled refugees from these regions, in addition to testing all patients who present with nausea, jaundice, and/or fatigue (**Fig. 3**). Most of the time the clinician should screen on arrival for chronic hepatitis B and C.

Although some refugees undergo screening overseas with surface antigen for hepatitis B before vaccination, no uniform overseas migration programs currently screen for these diseases, and so it is an important role for the refugee clinician. Positive serologies for hepatitis B core antibody and hepatitis B surface antigen are markers of chronic infection.[20] These patients should undergo hepatic function testing, imaging (typically with ultrasound), and evaluation by a specialist. Serology positive for only hepatitis B core antibody can indicate a resolved infection, early acute infection, low-level chronic infection, or simply be a false positive. Serologies should be repeated along with a hepatitis B e-antibody and e-antigen with referral to specialty care as appropriate. Reese and colleagues further detail hepatitis B evaluation both overseas and during the initial domestic screening examination. Positive serology for hepatitis C should be sent for quantitative RNA measurement. If hepatitis C RNA is detected, evaluation for underlying chronic liver disease and treatment is recommended[21].

Intestinal Parasites

Intestinal parasites are endemic in many regions of the world. Thanks to the Canadian immigrant and refugee guidelines,[1] we know that most parasites will disappear once the refugee has left the endemic area.[1] This allows clinicians to forgo stool testing for ova and parasites and culture and sensitivity, except in symptomatic patients. The 2 parasites that can persist, and cause serious harm up to 50 years later, are schistosomiasis and strongyloides; both are amenable to serology screening and treatment.[10]

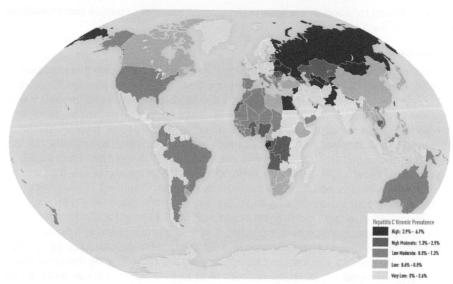

Fig. 3. Countries most affected by hepatitis C. (*From* Spradling P. Hepatitis C. In: Brunette GW, Nemhauser JB, editors. CDC health information for international travel 2020. New York: Oxford University Press; 2019; with permission.)

Treatment is relatively straight forward, with short courses of praziquantel and ivermectin or albendazole, respectively. Reese and colleagues provide detailed information about testing and treatment of common parasitic infections.

OTHER EMERGING INFECTIOUS DISEASES RELEVANT FOR IMMIGRANTS AND REFUGEES

Clinicians should focus on the list of infectious diseases listed earlier, which are associated with evidence-based screening and treatment. Immigrants and refugees are coming from around the world and a range of living conditions, and this increases disease exposure and the possibility of arrival with other tropical diseases. Clinicians should remain alert to diagnose, but not routinely screen, the following list of emerging diseases.

Malaria

Malaria, a blood born parasite, continues to kill millions of people around the world.[22] Spread via the *Anopheles* mosquito, there are five forms of *Plasmodium* that may be transmitted to humans, with the most common being *Plasmodium falciparum, Plasmodium vivax, and Plasmodium ovale.* Maps have emerged that show that even in tropical African cities, infections and deaths can vary dramatically within postal codes.[23] Most Western travelers will not spend time in neighborhoods with stagnant water and sewage, lack of air conditioning, and inadequately treated malaria, all risk factors for infection. Refugees, however, may come from high-risk malaria zones, and initiatives from the CDC have led to preemptive treatment at the time of migration to prevent malaria during travel.[8] Research has shown that a small portion of refugees will become sick with malaria after arrival, and Canadian guidelines recommend thick and thin smear for malaria when fever and fatigue within 3 months of arrival suggest a need for diagnosis.[1] Rapid diagnostic test may also be useful in remote towns that do not have access to blood smear testing. Treatment requires expertise and immediate consultation.[22]

Chikungunya

Chikungunya is endemic to countries in Africa, Asia, and Europe and more recently in the Americas and Caribbean. It is transmitted primarily through 2 species of mosquitoes, *Aedes aegypti* and *Aedes albopictus*, although blood-borne and in-utero transmission is also possible.[24] The hallmarks of chikungunya are a severe fever and arthralgia.[25] Other symptoms include nausea/vomiting, headache, myalgia, conjunctivitis, and maculopapular rash. Complications include myocarditis, hepatitis, hemorrhage, and ocular and nervous conditions among others.[26] In most patients, resolution of symptoms is seen within 10 days of symptom onset. Although arthralgia may persist for months to years in certain patients, mortality is rare. Diagnosis is usually clinical and based on travel exposure; diagnostic tests are done through testing for the virus (culture), viral RNA, or antibodies (immunoglobulin M). Treatment is supportive and focuses on symptom management, including fluids, acetaminophen, and nonsteroidal antiinflammatory drugs. Disease-modifying antirheumatic drugs, such as methotrexate can be used for the management of chronic arthritis following the initial infection. Such prolonged symptomatic courses tend to be seen in older patients, those with severe acute disease and underlying osteoarthritis. Precautions should be taken to avoid further transmission of the virus from the patient by avoiding further mosquito bites. No vaccine exists for chikungunya; prevention mostly consists of mosquito protection including applied repellant, screens, and clothing that covers most skin surfaces.[25] Clinicians caring for immigrants, refugees, migrant workers, and other travellers should remain alert for this new disease.

Chagas

Chagas, a disease caused by the parasitic protozoa *Trypanosoma cruzi* is thought to affect close to 8 million people primarily in Central and South America.[26] The parasite is transmitted through the triatomine bug, which frequents thatched-roof housing. Following a blood meal, *T cruzi*, which passes through the triatomine gut and into its excrements, is able to penetrate the human skin through the resultant bite marks. Chagas disease has an initial acute phase of 8 to 12 weeks, where infected individuals remain largely asymptomatic or experience nonspecific symptoms. After this period, the parasite levels found in blood drop to undetectable levels. At this point, the virus enters its chronic phase. It may take 1 of 2 forms. In the indeterminate form patients experience no symptoms, whereas the determinate form is characterized by cardiomyopathy and gastrointestinal disease.[26] Cardiomyopathy will develop in 20% to 30% of those with the indeterminate form and will result in various presentations, including heart failure and arrhythmias. The 10% to 15% who will develop gastrointestinal disease experience esophageal motility issues or colonic dilatation. The mainstay of treatment of the indeterminate form of Chagas is antitrypanosomal medications (benznidazole and nifurtimox). Monitoring for cardiac and intestinal complications is also recommended.

Endemic countries have seen a reduction in the incidence of the disease due to various factors including programs to reduce vector transmission in endemic areas and migration from rural to urban areas in Latin America. Chagas has significant implications for host countries, including congenital, transfusion and transplant transmission, and the management of associated comorbidities by health care practitioner.[27] The screening of refugees for Chagas disease is not routine at this time in the United States, although there is some indication that screening in targeted populations may be advantageous.[8] Most individuals will present with intestinal or cardiac symptoms.

Scabies

Scabies has reemerged as a prevalent concern in the context of large numbers of migrating and traveling people. Individuals living in crowded, close conditions such as refugee camps, schools, and elderly care facilities are at risk for contracting the scabies parasite, *Sarcoptes scabiei*.[28] Remain alert for this parasite, with its hallmark severe nocturnal itch and location in the interdigital, abdomen, and leg areas. The treatment is topical permethrin. Chronic scabies is a more challenging diagnosis; it often include multiagent infection with staphylococcus and even yeast contamination. Approaches to chronic scabies should address impetigo, scabies, yeast, and contact dermatitis when suspected, and follow-up in 2 weeks to consider additional treatment as needed.

Sexually Transmitted Infections

A host of sexually transmitted infections (STIs) remain a concern for many migrant and nonmigrant population. Some governments, such as Canada, Australia, and New Zealand, have included syphilis—Venereal Disease Research Laboratory—testing and penicillin treatment as part of their overseas migration screening process.[1,8,9] The United States (CDC) has its own guidance, which includes screening and treatment of syphilis and gonorrhea overseas.[29] Refugees who test positive for syphilis or gonorrhea are offered HIV testing. Other countries, such as United Kingdom, European Union, and Canada, have integrated immigrant and refugee STI testing within primary health care and public health systems.

SUMMARY

Clinicians who care for immigrants and refugees now have several national and international resources to prioritize and treat infectious diseases. Many of the familiar diseases remain in the screening list including interferon-gamma release assay or tuberculin skin test for latent TB followed by treatment. In addition, blood serology for HIV and hepatitis B and C provides accurate screening and allows clinicians to consider early treatment for better long-term outcomes. A newcomer on the list is serology for intestinal parasites, strongyloides and schistosomiasis, as both of these parasites may cause morbidity and mortality for up to 50 years. Current approaches use evidence and clinical decision support tools to guide clinicians and to improve the overall acceptability and feasibility and fairness of screening and treatment. Additional infectious diseases that warrant clinical alertness, if not actually screening, on the part of clinicians include malaria, chikungunya, Chagas, scabies, and COVID-19.

CLINICS CARE POINTS

- Latent TB now may be treated with either traditional INH or shorter-course rifampin or combination therapy.
- Community-based rapid HIV testing may improve uptake and access to results, counseling, and treatment.
- Serology testing for chronic and potentially harmful intestinal parasites has removed the need for routine stool testing for ova and parasites.
- Other infectious diseases that may sometimes warrant attention, based on symptoms, include malaria, chikungunya, Chagas, scabies, and COVID-19.

DISCLOSURE

The authors have nothing to disclose.

REFERENCES

1. Pottie K, Greenaway C, Feightner J, et al. Evidence-based clinical guidelines for immigrants and refugees. CMAJ 2011;183(12):E824–925.
2. Mota L, Mayhew M, Grant KJ, et al. Rejecting and accepting international migrant patients into primary care practices: A mixed method study. Int J Migr Health Soc Care 2015;11(2):108–29.
3. Beach MC, Gary TL, Price EG, et al. Improving health care quality for racial/ethnic minorities: A systematic review of the best evidence regarding provider and organization interventions. BMC Public Health 2006;6:1–11.
4. Sackett DL, Rosenberg J, Gray M, et al. Evidence based practice: what it is and what it isn't. BMJ 1996;312(7023):71–2.
5. Masic I, Miokovic M, Muhamedagic B. Evidence based medicine - new approaches and challenges. Acta Inform Med 2008;16(4):219.
6. Alonso-Coello P, Oxman AD, Moberg J, et al. GRADE Evidence to Decision (EtD) frameworks: a systematic and transparent approach to making well informed healthcare choices. 2: Clinical practice guidelines. BMJ 2016;353:i2089.
7. Pottie K, Greenaway C, Hassan G, et al. Caring for a newly arrived Syrian refugee family. CMAJ 2016. https://doi.org/10.1503/cmaj.151422.
8. Centers for Disease Control and Prevention, National Center for Emerging and Zoonotic Infectious Diseases (NCEZID) D of GM and Q (DGMQ). Guidelines for the U.S. Domestic Medical Examination for Newly Arriving Refugees. Available at: https://www.cdc.gov/immigrantrefugeehealth/guidelines/domestic/domestic-guidelines.html. Accessed July 28, 2019.
9. Chaves NJ, Paxton GA, Biggs BA, et al. The Australasian Society for Infectious Diseases and Refugee Health Network of Australia recommendations for health assessment for people from refugee-like backgrounds: an abridged outline. Med J Aust 2017;206(7):310–5.
10. European Centre for Disease Prevention and Control. Public health guidance on screening and vaccination for infectious diseases in newly arrived migrants within the EU/EEA. Stockholm (Sweden): ECDC; 2018.
11. Migration Health and Development Research Initiative. MHADRI. Available at: https://migrationhealthresearch.iom.int/mhadri. Accessed July 28, 2019.
12. Andrews JC, Schünemann HJ, Oxman AD, et al. GRADE guidelines: 15. Going from evidence to recommendation - Determinants of a recommendation's direction and strength. J Clin Epidemiol 2013;66(7):726–35.
13. Migrant Workers Alliance for Change. Unheeded warnings: COVID-19 and migrant workers in Canada. June 2020. Available at: https://migrantworkersalliance.org/wp-content/uploads/2020/06/Unheeded-Warnings-COVID19-and-Migrant-Workers.pdf. Accessed October 31, 2020.
14. Kluge HHP, Jakab Z, Bartovic J, et al. Refugee and migrant health in the COVID-19 response. Lancet 2020;395(10232):1237–9.
15. Worthman J, Lee J, Althomson S. Characteristics of persons who died with COVID-19 — United States, February 12–May 18, 2020. MMWR Morb Mortal Wkly Rep 2020;69:923–9.
16. Shea KM, Kammerer JS, Winston CA, et al. Estimated rate of reactivation of latent tuberculosis infection in the United States, overall and by population subgroup. Am J Epidemiol 2014;179:216–25.

17. Sterling TR, Njie G, Zenner D, et al. Guidelines for the Treatment of Latent Tuberculosis Infection: Recommendations from the National Tuberculosis Controllers Association and CDC, 2020. MMWR Recomm Rep 2020;69(No. RR-1):1–11.

18. Pottie K, Lotfi T, Kilzar L, et al. The effectiveness and cost-effectiveness of screening for HIV in migrants in the EU/EEA: A systematic review. Int J Environ Res Public Health 2018;15(8):1700.

19. Pottie K, Medu O, Welch V, et al. Effect of rapid HIV testing on HIV incidence and services in populations at high risk for HIV exposure: An equity-focused systematic review. BMJ Open 2014;4(12). https://doi.org/10.1136/bmjopen-2014-006859.

20. Centers for Disease Control and Prevention. Recommendations for Identification and Public Health Management of Persons with Chronic Hepatitis B Virus Infection. MMWR 2008;57(No. RR-8):1–20.

21. Wilkins T, Akhtar M, Gititu E, et al. Diagnosis and management of hepatitis C. Am Fam Physician 2015;91(12):835–42.

22. Guidelines for the treatment of malaria. 3rd edition. Geneva (Switzerland): World Health Organization; 2015. Available at: https://www.ncbi.nlm.nih.gov/books/NBK294440/. Accessed December 3, 2020.

23. FerrariG, Ntuku HM, Schmidlin S, et al. A malaria risk map of Kinshasa, Democratic Republic of Congo. Malar J 2016;15:27.

24. Centers for Disease Control and Prevention. CDC Yellow Book 2020: health information for international travel. New York: Oxford University Press; 2017.

25. World Health Organization. Chikungunya. Available at: https://www.who.int/newsroom/fact-sheets/detail/chikungunya. Accessed December 3, 2020.

26. Strickland G, Thomas, ed. Hunter's Tropical Medicine and emerging infectious diseases 8th ed. Philadelphia, W.B. Saunders Company 2000. 1102p. ilus. https://doi.org/10.1590/S0036-46652001000200018

27. Lidani KCF, Andrade FA, Bavia L, et al. Chagas disease: From discovery to a worldwide health problem. J Phys Oceanography 2019;49(6):1–13.

28. Brunette GW, Nemhauser JB. CDC Yellow Book 2020: health information for international travel. Oxford, England: Oxford University Press; 2020. Available at: https://wwwnc.cdc.gov/travel/yellowbook/2020/travel-related-infectious-diseases/scabies. Accessed December 3, 2020.

29. Centers for Disease Control and Prevention. Panel Physicians Technical Instructions. 2017. Available at: https://www.cdc.gov/immigrantrefugeehealth/exams/ti/panel/technical-instructions-panel-physicians.html. December 3, 2020.

Impact of COVID-19 on Resettled Refugees

Micah Brickhill-Atkinson, Fern R. Hauck, MD, MS, FAAFP*

KEYWORDS

- COVID-19 • Refugees • Vulnerable populations • Health care access

KEY POINTS

- Refugees experience unique challenges during the COVID-19 pandemic, including suspension of resettlement.
- Other harms of COVID-19 that affect the population at large have intensified effects on refugees, such as economic and disease vulnerability, mental illness exacerbations, communication challenges, and educational disruption.
- The Society of Refugee Healthcare Providers published guidelines for assessing refugees' barriers to following COVID-19 preventive recommendations.
- Recent reports from refugee health care providers offer suggestions for mitigating pandemic-related harm, including communication, case management, and advocacy.

INTRODUCTION

The novel coronavirus SARS-CoV-2 (COVID-19) has infected nearly 13 million people and has caused more than 570,000 deaths globally.[1] As the pandemic creates new challenges for worldwide communities, the refugee crisis remains another of humanity's grave tragedies. Refugees displaced due to war, violence, and oppression number 21.3 million worldwide.[2] As of April 4, 2020, thirty-four countries with substantial refugee resettlement reported local COVID-19 transmission.[3] Statistical data about the impact of COVID-19 on this population is scarce,[4] but a growing body of literature reveals that bureaucracy, poverty, and discrimination have threatened the well-being of refugees during the pandemic.[2] COVID-19 has additionally highlighted barriers to accessing health care for refugees,[5] who stand foremost among the world's most vulnerable people. The United Nations 2030 Agenda for Sustainable Development contains a promise to ensure no one is left behind,[3] and COVID-19 will only be controlled when all populations are included in the response.[5] Current literature

Department of Family Medicine, University of Virginia, PO Box 800729, Charlottesville, VA 22908-0729, USA
* Corresponding author.
E-mail address: frh8e@virginia.edu

Prim Care Clin Office Pract 48 (2021) 57–66
https://doi.org/10.1016/j.pop.2020.10.001
0095-4543/21/© 2020 Elsevier Inc. All rights reserved.

highlights 6 themes of the refugee pandemic experience (**Table 1**) and elucidates techniques for assessing barriers and alleviating harms.

SUSPENSION OF RESETTLEMENT AND RELATED SERVICES

Case 1: A.N. is a 30-year-old man from Afghanistan. He arrived in the United States 1 year ago. Soon after, his marriage to an Afghan woman was finalized, and he was assured that his wife would follow him to the United States. Now, he reports significant anxiety after his wife's migration was delayed due to COVID-19. The couple was informed that reunification would be deferred for at least 6 months.

Kathleen Newland of the Migration Policy Institute aptly pronounces, "COVID-19 has been the greatest disruption to human movement since World War II."[6] On March 10, 2020, the International Organization for Migration and the United Nations High Commissioner for Refugees (UNHCR) suspended refugee resettlement in the wake of worldwide travel restrictions.[7] The hold was lifted on June 18, 2020, after 10,000 refugee migrations were deferred. Some travel restrictions remain in place and continue to delay life-saving departures for persecuted people.[8] In addition, downstream effects such as expiration of security checks and overseas health examinations postpone travel for months after the resumption of resettlement.[9] Displaced persons are at risk of persecution in their countries of origin, and families face prolonged separation. Precedents from Ebola and SARS show that travel bans additionally incite stigma for migrant communities already in host countries.[10] Suspensions tend to harm refugees without benefiting host countries because many migrants would travel from an unaffected country to a nation with already high case counts. According to a World Health Organization report in 2018, refugees are at a low risk of transferring communicable disease to the host population in general.[7]

Table 1
Impacts of COVID-19 on resettled and accepted refugees

Suspension of Resettlement and Related Services	• Prolonged persecution • Delayed reunification • Expiration of security and health checks • Modified resettlement assistance after arrival
Economic Hardship	• Disproportionate job loss • Difficulty accessing relief • Reduced support for overseas family members
Disease Vulnerability	• Overcrowded living conditions • Comorbidities • High risk occupations • Delayed care and public health measures
Mental Illness Exacerbations	• Higher need • Memories of forced isolation and hiding • Modified and reduced mental health services
Communication Challenges	• Need for linguistically appropriate information • Barriers to virtual communication
Pediatric Impacts	• Boredom and loss of daily structure • School closings

Newly arrived refugees also face reduced volunteer and public services during the pandemic.[7] Volunteers and staff may be quarantined or restricted by government mandates, which disturbs provision of resettlement resources.[2] For example, the International Rescue Committee (IRC) in Charlottesville, Virginia typically provides an orientation for refugees attending their first medical appointment. Staff members transport clients to the family medicine clinic and show them how to find the waiting room and register. COVID-19 restrictions do not allow such transportation or accompaniment, and refugees must navigate the unfamiliar health system alone (E. Uhlmann, MPH, personal communication, July 16, 2020).

ECONOMIC HARDSHIP

> *Case 2*: M.K. is a 35-year-old single mother of four. She and her daughters arrived in the United States 2 years ago, and she began working as a hotel housekeeper. She lost her job during COVID-19 and has not found new employment. Her landlord comes to the apartment for rent, evoking tremendous anxiety. The family fears eviction as funds become scarce.

For resettled refugees, the impact of COVID-19 manifests in part through economic hardship. Migrant groups tend to fill difficult, low-paying occupations in their host countries.[4] In a study of 8 nations that house more than one-third of the world's refugee population, refugees were 60% more likely to lose jobs or income due to COVID-19 than the local population. About 60% worked in the most affected occupations, such as food services and retail, compared with 37% of the host population.[11] Low-income households have less ability to work remotely, which creates increased susceptibility to job loss amid the pandemic.[12] Refugees often carry the additional burden of sending money to family in their country of origin, so pandemic-related economic hardship reaches even further than those immediately affected by job loss.[6] Refugees also face barriers in accessing public services and safety nets. The Kovler Center Child Trauma Program (KCCTP), which serves refugee families in Chicago, recently noted that families frequently experienced job loss and struggled to access unemployment benefits.[13]

DISEASE VULNERABILITY

> *Case 3*: N.D., her husband, and 5 children are refugees living in an apartment with 1 bathroom. Even prepandemic, sharing a bathroom caused problems such as constipation in one of the children due to withholding bowel movements. COVID-19 measures seem nearly impossible to the family in light of their crowded home.

COVID-19's disease burden is higher in low-income settings such as resettled refugee populations due to living conditions, comorbidities, high-risk jobs, and delayed care and public health measures. The London School of Hygiene and Tropical Medicine reports that large and multigenerational households are a major reason for the disproportionate impact.[12] Overcrowded housing confers an increased risk of contracting disease,[7] and refugees often live in conditions that make hygiene and distancing impossible.[5] Management of chronic illnesses, such as diabetes mellitus and human immunodeficiency virus (HIV), is especially challenging among refugee populations during the pandemic.[14] Patients may be afraid to leave the house and may not be able to access prescriptions or appointments.

Endale and colleagues[13] propose that refugees are disproportionately affected by COVID-19 due to the frequency of high-risk jobs. For example, a high proportion of African refugees in the United States fill nursing home caretaker roles, which places them in one of the most vulnerable settings.[15] Low-income families are disincentivized from infection control measures, such as staying home from work, because their livelihoods are stretched too far.[12]

Refugees are vulnerable to stigma about disease transmission, which may make them fearful to disclose symptoms.[15] They may also delay seeking care due to fears of contagion or loss of legal protection.[10] In addition, widespread testing and contact tracing are less feasible in low-income settings; therefore, the current extent of disease is likely underestimated.[12]

MENTAL ILLNESS EXACERBATIONS

Case 4: S.A. is a 25-year-old female refugee with depression, anxiety, and posttraumatic stress disorder (PTSD) who presents to clinic with a chief concern of "stomach pain." During the interview, she becomes tearful as she describes increased nightmares and feeling hopeless when she thinks of her family members still in her country of exit. She fears leaving her apartment and contracting COVID-19, which evokes memories of forced hiding in her childhood.

Mental health is a chief concern among refugees during both pre- and post-pandemic circumstances. Systematic reviews estimate prevalences of up to 44% for anxiety, 44% for depression, and 36% for PTSD.[2] Migrants are more vulnerable to mental health risks in pandemics than the host population.[13] A 2020 literature review of international journals examined factors that worsen refugee mental health and found substantial commonality with risk factors for COVID-19.[2] Overlapping themes included overcrowding; disrupted sewage disposal; lower standards of hygiene; poor nutrition; reduced sanitation; and lack of shelter, health care, public services, and safety.[2] Boredom, isolation, inadequate supplies, lack of information, financial concerns, and disease-related stigma exacerbate the psychosocial effects of pandemics and quarantine.[13] Isolation and lack of control, prominent conditions in the COVID-19 setting, are known to exacerbate PTSD. Memories of forced hiding may be evoked by lockdowns and empty streets, and the pandemic may be reminiscent of Ebola and cholera for African migrants.[15]

Host countries face overloaded mental health care at baseline, making them ill equipped to adequately care for the pandemic-induced exacerbations among refugees.[2] Community-based mental health resources have moved to remote operations, making access even more difficult.[13] Baseline shortages combined with the exacerbating factors of a pandemic set up an environment for crisis among refugee mental health patients.

COMMUNICATION CHALLENGES

Case 5: D.N. is a 30-year-old female refugee from Afghanistan who recently arrived to the United States. She has a history of domestic abuse and fled her husband's family with her 3 children. In the few months since her arrival, she presented to clinic four times with vague somatic concerns, anxiety, and depressed mood. She was offered telephone therapy, as the clinic had paused in-person counseling sessions due to the health system's COVID-19 precautions. However, she is reluctant to share her traumatic experiences over the phone and reports little benefit from these sessions. She asks if she can instead participate in in-person therapy, where she would feel more comfortable discussing her trauma history.

Communication is a particular challenge for refugee patients in the pandemic setting. Lau and colleagues remind providers that communication is especially important for displaced populations who distrust authorities because of past experiences.[10] One challenge arises in accessible information sharing. Refugees struggle to find culturally and linguistically appropriate data about COVID-19.[7] Obstacles also present in the arena of telecommunication. The KCCTP noted the following barriers to refugee telemedicine: computer and Internet access; technological proficiency; attention span; decreased speed of interpretation; and privacy concerns.[13] Shared living conditions and unstable housing make private virtual communication difficult for many families. Providers at the Boston Center for Refugee Health and Human Rights (BCRHHR) noted that patients were sometimes unwilling to share trauma or torture histories over phone or video.[15] Although the host population may rely on virtual information sharing, refugees face added barriers in accessing these alterative communication modalities.

PEDIATRIC IMPACTS

Case 6: C.K. and M.K. are 7-year-old twins who arrived to the United States 1 year ago. In clinic, it is noted that they speak and understand little English. Their mother relates that they cannot read in any language. They do not speak English at home, and they did not attend school the past 4 months due to closings.

Pediatric refugees' daily functioning has suffered during COVID-19, attributable to boredom, isolation, and loss of daily structure.[13] IRC Medical Case Manager Erica Uhlmann in Charlottesville, Virginia notes a pattern of refugee parents overprotecting their children and prohibiting them from going outside. The IRC and partnering medical providers are educating families that time outside is safe and healthy as long as social distance is maintained (E. Uhlmann, MPH, personal communication, July 16, 2020).

School closings detrimentally affect refugee children. A systematic review of factors influencing pediatric refugee mental health found that schooling is essential for their adaptation and positive mental health. A sense of belonging at school is associated with lower PTSD and higher self-esteem, whereas lack of school attendance correlates with externalizing behavior. Poor connectedness with a school increases risk of depression, anxiety, and somatic stress.[16] Schools also provide a vital role in language acquisition for recently resettled children. Refugee students of all ages learn academic English in 4 to 7 years under ideal circumstances, but the interval increases to 10 years with interruptions to formal education. Schools maintain an indispensable role for educating migrant students and reducing achievement disparities.[17] Although distance learning may be accessible for some students, limited technological proficiency among refugee families poses a barrier to remote schooling.[13] The isolating conditions created by COVID-19 may have devastating impacts on pediatric refugee health and development.

TECHNIQUES TO ASSESS BARRIERS

The Society of Refugee Healthcare Providers issued guidelines to assess resettled refugees' barriers to following COVID-19 preventive behaviors. These include questions about fear of stigma or discrimination (eg, How have others in your community acted toward those who have become sick?); disease understanding (eg, Can you tell me about the symptoms of COVID-19?); how the patient communicates with providers and accesses information (eg, Before the pandemic, how did you normally communicate with your health care provider?); difficulties with prevention recommendations (eg, Do you have face masks, soap, hand sanitizer, etc.?); barriers to health care (eg, Do you know where to go for COVID-19 testing?); and social support (eg, Is there someone you can call if you need assistance with groceries, medications, or other essential needs if you become sick?).[18] The full assessment is available in **Box 1**.

TECHNIQUES TO MITIGATE HARMS

Refugee providers have published recommendations for reducing the harms of COVID-19. The BCRHHR issued the following suggestions: provide weekly email blasts about available community resources; watch for PTSD reemerging out of remission; remain mindful of patients' tolerance and attention span in telehealth sessions and consider shorter sessions if needed; maintain flexibility with in-person visits if patients are uncomfortable over the phone, especially patients who dissociate; and know the area's concrete food bank, unemployment, and shelter resources.[15]

The KCCTP offered the following resources to migrant families: exercise videos; guided relaxation and meditation; educational activities; caregiver guides; peer group video calls; virtual storybook readings; and cognitive behavioral therapy. The organization also initiated a response termed "Psychological First Aid." The approach started with information dissemination, dedicating attention to language accessibility. Next, providers turned their focus to active outreach, extensive case management, and telemedicine services.[13] The University of Virginia International Family Medicine Clinic similarly prioritized information dissemination and mailed handouts from the Centers for Disease Control and Prevention (CDC) to families in their first languages (Fern R. Hauck, MD, MS, personal communication, July 21, 2020). Multilingual print resources from the CDC can be found at the following Web address: https://wwwn.cdc.gov/pubs/other-languages. The UNHCR found that digital communication techniques are also useful for sharing information with refugees.[2]

Fawad and colleagues discuss the unique challenges of refugee chronic disease management in a pandemic.[14] The 2009 H1N1 influenza outbreak demonstrated the need for contingency planning in chronic disease management; deaths from stroke, myocardial infarction, and acute heart failure increased in this epidemic setting. Providers may consider extended medication supplies, especially for heart disease, HIV, tuberculosis, and contraception.[10]

Policy-level mitigation can also help alleviate harms for refugees during COVID-19. For example, public health leaders in the United Kingdom call for temporary citizenship rights for all migrant groups.[4] The UNHCR recommends full health care service access for refugees, reminding leaders that protecting all members ultimately shields the community at large.[10] The Center for Global Development advocates for fast-track credentialing of refugees who could contribute to the nation's health response or assist with personal protective equipment manufacturing, contact tracing, and delivery services. Allocating COVID-19 relief money to local nongovernmental organizations is another strategy to meet refugee needs. Currently, only 0.07% of US COVID-19 relief funds reach these nonprofit agencies that have a record of effective local community service.[11]

Local and national leaders, providers, and neighbors can also mitigate harm by maintaining a posture of openness and trust. Lessons from Ebola and SARS offer reminders that engaging communities and building trust contribute to the achievement of public health measures, whereas stigmatization opposes success. Transparency, trust, and community partnership are essential for disease control.[10]

Box 1
Society of Refugee Healthcare Providers Guide to Assessing Barriers to Following COVID-19 Prevention Guidance Among Resettled Refugees

Patient Communication
1. Before the COVID-19 pandemic, how did you normally communicate with your health care provider?
2. Did you use an interpreter to communicate with your health care provider?
3. What is your preferred method of communication with health care providers? (eg, email, telephone, text messaging, mailed letter, direct provider interaction)
   a. *If text message, mail, email, or telephone:* do you have anyone who can interpret (verbal) or translate (nonverbal, ie, documents) for you if needed? If so, is it a professional interpreter, community member, friend, or family member?
   b. *If the interpreter was a community member, friend, or family:* have you felt fear or embarrassment when someone other than a professional interpreter was used to discuss health conditions?
4. How do you access information about COVID-19? (eg, Internet, television, newspaper, friends, social group, faith-based group, social media such as WhatsApp, TikTok)

Patient Understanding of COVID-19
1. Can you tell me about the symptoms of COVID-19?
2. Can you tell me about some health complications of COVID-19?
3. How do you protect yourself from getting sick with COVID-19?
4. How do you prevent family members and others from getting sick with COVID-19?
5. How would you normally treat *[list symptoms that are currently associated with COVID-19]*:
   a. Fever?
   b. Dry Cough?
   c. Fatigue?
   d. Headache?
   e. Aches and pains?
   f. Sore throat?
   g. Chest pain?
   h. Difficulty breathing or shortness of breath?

Fear of Stigma or Discrimination
1. Do you know anyone in your community who has either become sick with COVID-19 or tested positive for COVID-19?
2. How have others in your community acted toward those who have become sick?
3. Would you communicate with someone who was diagnosed with COVID-19? If so, how? When would you resume meeting the person face-to-face?

Barriers to Following COVID-19 Prevention Recommendations
1. Is there any person in your home who can help with household responsibilities if you were to become sick? *[this is primarily asked to persons living with others, such as adults and children].*
2. If someone in your house was to get sick with COVID-19, do you have a way to keep a six feet distance from other household members within your house?
3. Are you or anyone else in your household currently working?
   a. If yes:
      i. where are you/they working?
      ii. what information has your/their employer provided?
      iii. what steps have your/their employer taken to keep you and your family safe?
      iv. If you or someone in your household were to become sick with COVID-19, do you think you would be able to miss work until you or your family member feel better and a medical professional said it was safe for you to go back to work?
   b. If no one in the household is currently working, what support are you receiving financially?
4. Do you have access to:
   a. Face masks and gloves?
   b. Soap and/or hand sanitizer?

    c. Household cleaners and disinfectants?
    d. Enough dishware, eating utensils, clothes, towels, and bedding for sick and healthy family members?
    e. Essential needs such as a food, medications, and basic amenities (eg, electricity)?

Barriers to Health Care Access
1. Do you know where to go to receive testing for COVID-19? If yes, how did you find out about the testing site?
2. Do you know where to go to receive health care for COVID-19?
3. How would you get to a health care facility if you were sick and needed to see a health care provider?
4. Can you describe when you would feel you need to call 911? Are you comfortable calling 911?
5. Do you have health insurance that can help support your health care needs if you get sick?
6. Is there any reason that would prevent you from seeking care if you become sick?

Available Social Support
1. Is there someone you can call to support you (and/or your family) if you become sick? If you need to go to the emergency room?
2. Do you think this person can continue to assist you if you were diagnosed with COVID-19?
3. Is there someone you can call if you need assistance with groceries, medications, laundry and/or other essential needs while you are sick?
4. Do you think this person can continue to assist you if you were diagnosed with COVID-19?

From Guide to Assessing Barriers to Following COVID-19 Prevention Guidance Among Resettled Refugees. New York: Society of Refugee Healthcare Providers; 2020. License: CC BY-NC-SA 4.0.; with permission.

SUMMARY

The novel coronavirus SARS-CoV-2 poses singular challenges to the world's resettled refugee population. Suspension of resettlement prolongs suffering for refugees accepted but not yet relocated and delays family reunification, and modified resettlement agency operations create challenges for new arrivals. Refugees are particularly vulnerable to both economic hardship and severe disease in the wake of the pandemic. Mental illnesses, prevalent among this population at baseline, are exacerbated by isolative and uncertain conditions. Communication challenges make the virtual world less accessible to resettled refugees, and children suffer the consequences of boredom and loss of school resources. Refugee providers can mitigate harms by comprehensively assessing barriers faced by their patients, providing accessible information, and advocating for policies that include vulnerable populations and promote trust.

CLINICS CARE POINTS

- Implement questions from the Society for Refugee Healthcare Providers Guide to assess refugee patients' needs during the pandemic.
- Watch for PTSD reemergence and other mental illness exacerbations.
- Review local resources to enable concrete recommendations for refugees and all patients in need during the challenging pandemic conditions.
- Offer linguistically appropriate information about COVID-19 and preventive measures.

ACKNOWLEDGMENTS

Special thanks to Erica Uhlmann, International Rescue Committee Charlottesville Medical Case Manager.

DISCLOSURE

The authors have nothing to disclose.

REFERENCES

1. World Health Organization. Coronavirus disease (COVID-19) Situation Report – 176. 2020. Available at: https://www.who.int/docs/default-source/coronaviruse/situation-reports/20200714-covid-19-sitrep-176.pdf. Accessed July 14, 2020.
2. Júnior JG, Sales JPD, Moreira MM, et al. A crisis within the crisis: The mental health situation of refugees in the world during the 2019 coronavirus (2019-nCoV) outbreak. Psychiatry Res 2020;288:113000. Available at: https://www.ncbi.nlm.nih.gov/pmc/articles/PMC7156944/. Accessed July 16, 2020.
3. The Lancet. COVID-19 will not leave behind refugees and migrants. Lancet 2020; 395(10230):1090.
4. Bhopal RS. COVID-19: Immense necessity and challenges in meeting the needs of minorities, especially asylum seekers and undocumented migrants. Public Health 2020;182:161–2.
5. Orcutt M, Patel P, Burns R, et al. Global call to action for inclusion of migrants and refugees in the COVID-19 response. Lancet 2020;395(10235):1482–3.
6. Newland K. Lost in transition. Science 2020;368(6489):343.
7. Kluge HHP, Jakab Z, Bartovic J, et al. Refugee and migrant health in the COVID-19 response. Lancet 2020;395(10232):1237–9.
8. Joint Statement: UN refugee chief Grandi and IOM's Vitorino announce resumption of resettlement travel for refugees. United Nations High Commissioner for Refugees website. 2020. Available at: https://www.unhcr.org/en-us/news/press/2020/6/5eeb85be4/joint-statement-un-refugee-chief-grandi-ioms-vitorino-announce-resumption.html. Accessed July 16, 2020.
9. Bhattacharya CB, Fisher B. Refugee Assistance During a Global Pandemic. *Sustaining Sustainability.* 2020. Available at: https://soundcloud.com/user-148611772/episode-12-refugee-assistance-during-a-global-pandemic-with-betsy-fisher. Accessed July 14, 2020.
10. Lau LS, Sarmari G, Moresky RT, et al. COVID-19 in humanitarian settings and lessons learned from past epidemics. Nat Med 2020;26:647–8.
11. Dempster H, Ginn T, Graham J, et al. Locked Down and Left Behind: The Impact of COVID-19 on Refugees' Economic Inclusion. Center for Global Development, Refugees International, and International Rescue Committee. 2020. Available at: https://www.refugeesinternational.org/reports/2020/7/6/locked-down-and-left-behind-the-impact-of-covid-19-on-refugees-economic-inclusion. Accessed July 16, 2020.
12. Dahab M, van Zandvoort K, Flasche S, et al. COVID-19 control in low-income settings and displaced populations: what can realistically be done? London School of Hygiene and Tropical Medicine website. 2020. Available at: https://www.lshtm.ac.uk/newsevents/news/2020/covid-19-control-low-income-settings-and-displaced-populations-what-can. Accessed July 16, 2020.
13. Endale T, Jean NS, Birman D. COVID-19 and refugee and immigrant youth: A community-based mental health perspective. Psychol Trauma 2020;12(S1):

S225–7. Available at: https://europepmc.org/article/med/32478552. Accessed July 16, 2020.

14. Fawad M, Rawashdeh F, Parmar PK, et al. Simple ideas to mitigate the impacts of the COVID-19 epidemic on refugees with chronic diseases. Confl Health 2020;14: 23. Available at: https://www.ncbi.nlm.nih.gov/pmc/articles/PMC7201387/. Accessed July 16, 2020.

15. Mattar S, Piwowarczyk LA. COVID-19 and U.S.-based refugee populations: Commentary. Psychol Trauma 2020;12(S1):S228–9. Available at: https://europepmc.org/article/med/32538665. Accessed July 16, 2020.

16. Fazel M, Reed RV, Panter-Brick C, et al. Mental health of displaced and refugee children resettled in high-income countries: risk and protective factors. Lancet 2012;379:266–82.

17. McNeely CA, Morland L, Doty SB, et al. How schools can promote healthy development for newly arrived immigrant and refugee adolescents: Research priorities. J Sch Health 2017;87(2):121–32.

18. Society of Refugee Healthcare Providers. Guide to Assessing Barriers to Following COVID-19 Prevention Guidance Among Resettled Refugees. 2020. Available at: http://refugeesociety.org/wp-content/uploads/2020/04/Guide-Assessing-Barriers-COVID-19-SRHP-June2020.pdf. Accessed July 16, 2020.

Common Hematologic, Nutritional, Asthma/Allergic Conditions and Lead Screening/ Management

Brittany DiVito, MPH, MSN, FNP-BC[a], Rachel Talavlikar, MD[b,c],
Sarah Seifu, MD, MS[d,*]

KEYWORDS

- Anemia • Nutrition • Vitamin deficiency • Allergic rhinitis • Asthma • Lead toxicity
- Refugee

KEY POINTS

- A CBC should be collected in all newly arrived immigrant and refugee adults and children.
- Iron deficiency anemia is not a complete diagnosis; the cause must be established.
- Dietary history is pivotal in understanding nutrition before and after arrival, and cultural/ religious practices.
- Allergy and asthma management should include comprehensive education that considers health literacy levels, language barriers, and uses demonstration.
- Elevated lead levels remain an ongoing problem in foreign-born children; current CDC guidelines recommend routine screening on arrival and scheduled follow-up for all children aged 6 months to 16 years and pregnant/lactating mothers.

HEMATOLOGIC
Background

Newly arrived immigrants and refugees present with a range of hematologic conditions that when identified and treated early, can improve the trajectory of their health and resettlement. These range from genetic conditions to acquired disease as a result of infections or nutritional deficiencies. The diagnosis must take into context not only where a person was born and has lived, but also their migration journey.[1–3]

[a] Department of Family Medicine, District Medical Group/Valleywise Health, Refugee Family & Internal Medicine Clinic, 2525 East Roosevelt Street, Phoenix, AZ 85004, USA; [b] Department of Family Medicine, Cumming School of Medicine, University of Calgary, Calgary, Alberta, Canada; [c] Mosaic Refugee Health Clinic, 433 Marlborough Way Northeast, #530, Calgary, Alberta T2A 5H5, Canada; [d] University of Virginia Department of Family Medicine, PO Box 800729, Charlottesville, VA 22908-0729, USA
* Corresponding author.
E-mail address: ss6gp@virginia.edu

Prim Care Clin Office Pract 48 (2021) 67–81
https://doi.org/10.1016/j.pop.2020.10.002
0095-4543/21/Published by Elsevier Inc.

This section focuses on the commonly seen presentations and etiologies in this population but the general differential for all presentations must always be considered.

Screening

Guidelines for the United States suggest a complete blood count (CBC) with differential on arrival for all newcomers, regardless of age or ethnicity.[1,4] In Canada it is recommended to screen women and children.[2,3] When an abnormality is found, further testing for targeted evaluation to identify cause can be ordered. Testing depends on initial clinical presentation and risk stratification and any prearrival treatments received but could include: iron studies, hemoglobinopathy screening, vitamin B_{12} levels, peripheral blood smear, parasitic testing, glucose-6-phosphaste-dehydrogenase (G6PD) screening, malaria, human immunodeficiency virus (HIV), hepatitis B, liver and renal function, and age-appropriate testing including colorectal screening and urinalysis.[1–5]

Etiology and Risk Factors

Anemia

Iron deficiency anemia Studies suggest that anywhere from 11% to 37% of newcomers are found to be anemic on arrival.[1,2,5] Risk factors include having lived in a refugee camp, in poverty, a country with predominantly vegetarian diet, or anywhere that conflict might have impacted supply chain or food delivery.[2,3,5,6] However, it is important to remember that iron deficiency itself is not a diagnosis; is it is a symptom, and the underlying cause must be established.[7]

In this population, nutritional deficiency and poor intake are common causes that improve once resettled; however, confounding diagnoses must also be considered.[2,3] Iron deficiency may also be a result of gastrointestinal malabsorption possibly caused by parasitic infection (helminths), malabsorption secondary to *Helicobacter pylori* infection, or lead toxicity. Deficiency may also be a result of increased blood loss caused by menstrual, gastrointestinal, or urinary tract losses. Multiparity and being a female of reproductive age are identified risk factors.[1–3]

Depending on the severity and cause, dietary modifications are recommended along with iron replacement. Oral preparations are first line with citrus to optimize absorption. Dosing depends on the initial iron deficit. Treatment duration is typically 3 to 6 months. Patient tolerance influences the format chosen. In pregnant women and children, it is important to ensure that treatment is efficacious, because prolonged deficiency can impact cognitive development. Where oral formulations are not tolerated or successful, then intravenous formulations are considered. Intramuscular formulations are not recommended for use because of side effects.[5,8,9]

Other nutritional anemias Vitamin B_{12} deficiency can result in a macrocytic anemia. Often overlooked, it is of particular importance in anyone presenting with neurologic symptoms, such as weakness, fatigue, ataxia, cognitive changes, or peripheral neuropathic symptoms. It is often seen in refugees from Bhutan and in pregnant women. Possible causes include poor intake, thyroid disease, chronic *H pylori* infection, tapeworm infection, medication use, and more rarely pernicious anemia.[3,6,8]

Folate deficiency also presents with a macrocytic anemia and should be suspected in those who have experienced chronic hemolysis, pregnancy, those with strict dietary limitations, or in alcohol use disorder.[3,10]

For deficiencies including vitamin B_{12} and folate, replacement is typically oral or parenteral. More rapid replacement is indicated for those with neurologic findings or in pregnancy. Note that folic acid replacement can mask vitamin B_{12} deficiency.[11,12]

Box 1
Substances to avoid with G6PD deficiency

- Analgesics/antipyretics
  - Acetanilide, aspirin, acetophenetidin, antipyrine, dipyrone, **phenazopyridine**

- Sulfa drugs
  - Sulfanilamide, sulphapyridine, sulfacetamide, sulfamethoxazole, sulfisoxazole

- Antimalarials
  - Aminoquinolines (amodiaquine, chloroquine), **primaquine**, pamaquine, pentaquine, quinacrine, quinine

- Antibiotics
  - Chloramphenicol, **dapsone**, furazolidone, nalidixic acid, **nitrofurantoin**, niridazole, para-aminosalicylic acid

- Miscellaneous
  - Aminopyrine (used in liver tests); dimercaprol (antidote); mestranol (contraceptive); **methylene blue** (antidote); probenecid (gout), prochlorperazine (antipsychotic, antiemetic, anxiety); quinidine (antiarrhythmic); synthetic vitamin K; toluidine blue; uricase. **rasburicase** (gout)

- Food/domestic
  - **Fava (broad) beans, naphthalene (mothballs, henna), isobutyl nitrate (Poppers drugs)**

Bolded substances are especially unsafe.

From Refugee Health YYC. Available at: https://www.refugeehealthyyc.ca/appendix#G6PDDeficiencyMapaswellasListofSubstancestoAvoidwithInformationCardTemplate. Accessed Sept 24 2020; with permission.

Eastern descent and Sephardic Jews, West Indians, Yemenites, and those from Greece.[17]

A diagnosis of exclusion, it is based on a persistent mild neutropenia in a patient with an appropriate ethnic background and without a history of recurrent infections. The neutrophils are functionally normally and there are few clinical consequences to having it. It is generally associated with neutrophil counts greater than 1.0×10^9/L. Neutrophil counts less than 0.5 require specialist review. For diagnosis, it is suggested to repeat a CBC at least twice separated by 2 weeks. A review of systems and investigation for other common causes of neutropenia must be done.[5]

Eosinophilia

The differential diagnosis for eosinophilia (absolute count >450 cells/μL) is broad; however, in newcomer populations there are key etiologies that should be investigated initially unless initial clinical presentation warrants otherwise. Eosinophilia suggests an immune response and when parasitic in origin, is caused by helminthic migration through tissue. The most common parasitic causes of eosinophilia in newcomers are schistosomiasis and strongyloidiasis; however, other infections include ascariasis, filariases, hookworm, and echinococcosis.[1,3,5,18] Nonparasitic causes in a newcomer population can include fungal infection, HIV, and infestations (scabies or myiasis). Reese and colleagues article "Refugee Medical Screening", describe the appropriate evaluation for new arrivals with eosinophilia, including testing strategies and treatment. If the work-up for parasites is negative and eosinophilia persists, a widened differential is considered including allergies, collagen vascular disease, malignancy, and medication.[3]

Thrombocytopenia

Immigrants and refugees who present with thrombocytopenia must be assessed for acute infections including malaria, typhoid, or dengue and HIV. If clinically well, then further investigation for splenomegaly is warranted because they may have had prior history of multiple episodes of malaria or other infections, such as schistosomiasis or visceral leishmaniasis. Beyond this, it is important to assess whether this finding is isolated or part of a pancytopenia with the usual work-up for this seen in a general population warranted. Nutritional deficiencies must also be investigated (vitamin B_{12}, folate).[1,3,19]

NUTRITION
Background

For refugee populations, nutritional inadequacy can come in the form of malnutrition, undernutrition, vitamin deficiency, and/or elevated body mass index. Malnutrition is often associated with the lack of nutrition or lack of food from the home country. Undernutrition is now more often seen because of the cost of food and food insecurity once they have arrived in the United States. Vitamin deficiencies most often include iron, vitamin B_{12}, vitamin D, and sequela of parasite infections. There is also growing concern about overweight/obesity among refugees resettling to developed countries.[20,21] This is partially explained by the "immigrant paradox," which suggests that subsequent generations and increased time in the United States can lead to increased obesity and poorer health outcomes.[22] Refugee populations are at heightened risk of complications from undernutrition (ie, developmental and cognitive delays) and overweight/obesity (ie, chronic medical conditions, such as diabetes mellitus, hypertension, and other cardiovascular conditions), and adequate screening and treatment is important.[23] There are also special considerations related to substance abuse (alcoholism), pediatrics, chronic disease, older adults, parasites, immigrant paradox, and obesity that are outside the scope of this article.

Etiology/Risk Factors

The condition of the home country and/or refugee camp does not always provide adequate nutrition for refugees. Food insecurity is a major risk factor before and after arrival to the United States; one study found that up to two-thirds of participating refugees are affected.[24,25] In addition, limited funding, lack of access to nutritious food, dental barriers and/or pain, and knowledge gaps can also be risk factors for nutritional inadequacy in refugees.

Screening

Domestic health screening should include an assessment of nutritional deficiencies. An initial examination should include dietary history and restrictions, past and present food insecurity, anthropometric measures, physical examination, and blood work (**Tables 2** and **3**).[23] For those with an elevated body mass index (overweight or obese), chronic disease screening should also be completed.

Treatment

Nutritional counseling is recommended; this includes discussing access to food and cooking facilities, cultural adjustment, and determination of state/federal benefits. It is also important to encourage increased physical activity. Education and targeted interventions are important to reinforce, especially in the first 2 to 5 years after resettlement. Targeted interventions should include culturally

Table 2
Screening for nutritional inadequacy

Screening Evaluation	History and Findings Suggesting Nutritional Deficiency
Dietary history	Dietary habits and restrictions (religious, cultural), food allergies, alcohol/substance use, nutritional deficiencies
Social history	Previous food insecurity and/or distress, history of limited consumption of foods (fruits, vegetables, and meat), supplemental intake, breastfeeding status, history of fractures or skeletal deformities
Anthropometric measures	Accurate measurements of weight, height, and body mass index (>2 y old)
Physical examination	Cardiac (flow murmur, tachycardia), musculoskeletal, neurologic, integumentary, endocrine (thyroid), dental, eye examination

sensitive counseling and adjustments of foods known and used by the populations rather than counseling based on a Western diet. It is also recommended that all children 6 months to 5 years are given a multivitamin with iron.[23,26] For children, undernutrition is defined as weight-for-height less than the fifth percentile; no improvement with 3 months is considered failure to thrive and warrants further evaluation.[20]

ASTHMA AND ALLERGY RELATED CONDITIONS
Background

Asthma and allergic rhinitis is associated with high morbidity and financial expenses, especially for refugee populations. Some studies suggest that immigrating from a less developed country can serve as a protective factor for asthma, allergic rhinitis, and eczema.[27] However, other systematic reviews have concluded that migrating to a more developed country increases the rate of chronic diseases over time, specifically asthma and allergic diseases.[28,29] Immigrant and refugee children are initially found to have a lower prevalence of allergic disease, but this prevalence rises after approximately 10 years to a level consistent with children in the United States.[30] This health paradox has been shown across different racial and ethnic groups immigrating throughout various areas of the world with the risk for asthma and allergy highest when immigration occurs in early childhood.[31] The cause of this is hypothesized and considers acculturation, obesity, stress, and tobacco use.[31] Overall, proper diagnosis and treatment is best achieved with culturally competent care.

Etiology/Risk Factors

Refugees are at particularly high risk of respiratory disease because of their premigration living conditions in refugee camps and less developed countries. These living conditions often result in increased exposure to biomass smoke, smoke from open stoves, and industrial pollution. These exposures can have an effect on lung function, temporary or permanent, and may result in respiratory dysfunction, such as chronic obstructive lung disease or even lung cancer.[32] Men are at greatest risk of chronic disease related to tobacco use, whereas women, children, and elderly are at greater risk of disease secondary to fuels from indoor/outdoor cooking.[32] Outdoor allergens from the environment (ie, trees, pollens, smoke) and indoor allergens (ie, dust mites) also put patients at higher risk of allergy and asthma symptoms.

Table 3
History and physical examination findings in children and adolescents and associated nutritional deficiencies

Nutrient Deficiency	High-Risk Groups	Cause	Signs and Symptoms	Potential Long-Term Effects
Severe undernutrition	Children, low socioeconomic status	Food insecurity, decreased appetite, chronic diarrhea	Emaciation, marasmus kwashiorkor	Physical and/or mental disability
Iron deficiency	6–24 mo old, breastfed infants >6 mo without iron supplementation, premenopausal women	Low dietary availability, teas and phytates, parasitic infections, hematologic disorders, other micronutrient deficiencies	Flow murmur, pallor	Infants: impaired psychomotor/brain development Adolescents: cognitive impairments Adults: fatigue, low productivity, impaired reproduction
Vitamin D	Dark skin, limited sun exposure, infants breastfeeding >6 mo without supplement, pregnant/lactating women, climate, malabsorption	Inadequate dietary intake of vitamin D and calcium, iron; limited skin exposure (including protective/religious clothing)	Bone pain, fractures or skeletal deformities, poor growth, muscle weakness, craniotabes, costochondral swelling, dental problems	Rickets, osteoporosis
Vitamin B$_{12}$	Bhutanese descent (B$_{12}$ deficiency), limited access to fortified foods/animal products (eggs, meat, milk, eggs, fish), history of Helicobacter pylori infection	Decreased dietary intake, intrinsic factor deficiency, chronic gastritis from H pylori	Neurologic: loss of proprioception/reflexes, ataxia, peripheral neuropathy, anosmia Nonspecific: fatigue, impaired concentration/memory, irritability, depression, constipation, weight loss Infants (rare): failure to thrive, movement disorder, developmental delays, pancytopenia	Degeneration of the spinal cord; psychiatric illness

	Risk factors	Cause	Signs/Symptoms	Severe manifestations
Vitamin A	More common in developing world (refugee camps generally provide vitamin A supplementation so at risk if not provided)	Decreased vitamin A supplementation (liver, fish oils, milk, eggs, vegetables)	Xerosis, Bitot spots, poor night vision	Permanent blindness Impaired: bone growth, immune response, organ development
Zinc	Plant-based and/or low-protein diet	Diet low in zinc (meat, fish, nuts), and high in corn	Dermatitis, diarrhea, stomatitis, loss of weight/appetite, impaired immune function, hair loss, taste abnormalities, lethargy	Growth retardation, delayed sexual maturation/impotence
Thiamine/B$_1$	Diet high in white rice, alcohol, poor food intake (mushrooms, seeds, fish, pork pecans, nuts), history of recurrent diarrhea	Poor intake, altered metabolism (fever, pregnancy, breastfeeding, liver disease, hyperthyroidism), gastrointestinal losses, food with thiaminases or antihistamine compounds	Loss of appetite, constipation, fatigue, irritability, memory loss, peripheral neuropathy, muscle weakness and pain, areflexia, foot drop (dropsy), tachycardia, heart failure	Beriberi: wet or dry
Vitamin B$_3$, niacin and tryptophan	Inadequate intake of niacin and/or tryptophan, often in South Asia where people eat millet with high leucine content, alcoholism	Decreased dietary intake (fish, poultry, pork, liver, mushrooms, peas, avocado, sunflower seeds), secondary deficiency	Diarrhea, stomatitis, anxiety, tremors, peripheral neuritis; less known about children	Pellagra, neurologic symptoms
Vitamin C	Chronic malnutrition, alcoholism, restrictive diets (low in fruits/vegetables)	Decreased dietary intake	Ecchymosis, petechiae, bleeding gums, hyperkeratosis, impaired wound healing, weakness, malaise, joint pain/swelling, edema, depression, neuropathy	Scurvy: symptoms related to impaired collagen synthesis
Iodine	Developing country without iodized salt, most often school-aged children	Diet low in seafood, sea salt, iodized table salt	Palpable goiter	Cretinism hypothyroidism, growth and developmental abnormalities

Table 4
Screening and treatment of allergic rhinitis and asthma

Diagnosis	Screening	Treatment
Allergic rhinitis	Screen based on symptoms and physical examination, specific IgE testing not indicated unless initial treatment failed	Treatment based on symptoms: second-generation antihistamine (ie, loratadine, cetirizine), nasal glucocorticoid (ie, fluticasone), nasal antihistamine[38]; preference for nonpharmacologic treatment may include nasal saline and avoidance of allergens
Asthma	Screen based on history, risk factors, symptoms and physical examination, pulmonary function test (spirometry), chest radiograph not indicated unless severe symptoms and/or other cause suspected, determine asthma severity classification	Treat per guidelines that include significant education, action plan, short-acting β-agonist as needed, low-dose inhaled glucocorticoid, see stepwise approach[42]

Screening/Treatment

All newly arrived refugees have a domestic health screening on arrival. Because of the prevalence of latent tuberculosis (TB), many refugees also have a TB test and/or chest radiograph. Patients should have a thorough review of systems, and those who complain of asthma or allergy symptoms should be further evaluated to establish the correct diagnosis after arrival (**Table 4**). It may take years for allergen exposure to develop into allergic rhinitis and this diagnosis should be considered in refugees who have been resettled for several years. Patients should also be screened on arrival and treated for other causes of chronic cough, such as tobacco use, TB, obstructive sleep apnea, chronic obstructive pulmonary disease, and gastroesophageal reflux disease.[31]

LEAD SCREENING
Background

Lead neurotoxicity, otherwise known as lead poisoning, occurs when exposure causes direct and indirect damage to the central nervous system. This damage is particularly devastating on children and adolescents, whose brains are still undergoing critical development. Long-term effects include cognitive impairment and mood disturbances. These are correlated with neuroanatomic changes within the prefrontal cortex and brain volume loss.[33] There is no known exposure to lead that is considered "safe," because lead serves no physiologic purpose. In fact, neurotoxic effects have been noted following exposure to "low" lead levels. As such, lead neurotoxicity is a significant public health concern.[34]

Before June 2012, the Centers for Disease Control and Prevention (CDC) designated a blood lead level of greater than or equal to 10 μg/dL the threshold that should prompt swift public health action. In June 2012, the CDC incorporated a recommendation made by the Advisory Committee on Childhood Lead Poisoning Prevention and decreased this threshold to greater than or equal to 5 μg/dL.[35]

Risk Factors and Etiology

The US National Health and Nutrition Examination Survey reported a decline in the prevalence of elevated blood lead level (EBLL) in children ages 1 to 5 years from a reported 88% in 1976 to 1980 ($\geq$10 μg/dL) to 2.6% in 2007 to 2010 ($\geq$5 μg/dL).[36] However, EBLL remains a continuing problem for foreign-born children who relocate to North America. Refugee status in and of itself is considered a risk factor for EBLL, because they are subject to preresettlement and/or postresettlement exposure to lead.

The World Health Organization cites common sources of lead exposure that affect refugee children preresettlement. These include lead in traditional medicines, such as topicals and cosmetics; lead solder in drinking-water systems; and contaminated soil that poisons food.[37] Acknowledging the extensive and unique sociocultural traditions of refugees across the globe allows clinicians to understand the role these customs play in influencing lead neurotoxicity and therefore neurodevelopment.

In the United States, common sources of lead toxicity include lead-based paints and lead-contaminated dust found within industrial and public buildings.[38] Although lead-based paint was banned in the late 1970s, socioeconomic status continues to disproportionately affect vulnerable populations, including refugees. Out of an estimated 890,000 children ages 1 to 5 with EBLL, 60% were on Medicaid per the National Health and Nutrition Examination Survey III conducted in 1991 to 1995.[39]

Screening and Treatment

In refugee children who are resettled in the United States, the CDC recommends initial blood lead testing in children ages 6 months to 16 years within 90 days of arrival. Regardless of initial screening results, repeat testing is recommended 3 to 6 months after placement into a permanent housing to help determine if any postresettlement exposure has occurred.[40] The CDC also recommends initial and follow-up screening of pregnant and lactating women.[39] Any elevated screening results, usually obtained by capillary tube, must be confirmed with blood drawn by venipuncture (**Table 5**). Once adequate testing and follow-up have been performed (**Table 6**), health care providers are expected to follow treatment protocols per CDC guidelines for any individuals with EBLL (**Table 7**).[40]

Lead and Anemia

Lead causes microcytosis and microcytic anemia by inhibiting heme synthesis and causing a higher rate of red blood cell turnover. As a heavy metal, lead also interferes with iron absorption, which affects the use of iron in heme production. In turn, iron deficiency causes microcytic anemia and increases the absorption of heavy metals (ie, lead and cadmium). Anemia is common in refugee children and may be of nutritious

Table 5	
CDC recommended schedule for obtaining a confirmatory venous sample	
Blood Lead Level (μg/dL)	**CDC Recommendations**
$\geq$5–9	1–3 mo
10–44	1 wk to 1 mo; more urgency with higher number
45–59	48 h
60–69	24 h
$\geq$70	ASAP

Adapted from Centers for Disease Control and Prevention (CDC). Childhood Lead Poisoning Prevention: Recommended Actions Based on Blood Lead Level. Available at: https://www.cdc.gov/nceh/lead/advisory/acclpp/actions-blls.htm. Accessed April 4 2020.

Table 6
CDC schedule for follow-up blood lead testing

BLL	Early Follow Up Testing	Later Follow Up Testing
≥5–9 µg/dL	3 mo	6–9 mo
10–44 µg/dL	1–3 mo	3–6 mo
45–59 µg/dL	1–3 mo	1–3 mo
60–69 µg/dL	2 wk to 1 mo	1 mo
≥70 µg/dL	ASAP	ASAP

Adapted from Centers for Disease Control and Prevention (CDC). Childhood Lead Poisoning Prevention: Recommended Actions Based on Blood Lead Level. Available at: https://www.cdc.gov/nceh/lead/advisory/acclpp/actions-blls.htm. Accessed April 4 2020.

Table 7
CDC recommendations for follow-up and case management of children based on confirmed blood lead levels

Blood Lead Level (µg/dL)	CDC Recommendations
<5	Assess nutrition status and developmental milestones. Provide anticipatory guidance. Follow-up testing at recommended interval.
5–9	Same as above. Obtain environmental exposure history and home investigation. Provide nutritional counseling regarding Ca2+ and iron.
10–19	Same as above. Consider laboratory work to asses iron status.
20–44	Same as above. Obtain history and physical for neurodevelopmental assessment. Assess iron status and hemoglobin/hematocrit. Obtain abdominal X-Ray.
45–69	Same as above. Complete neurologic examination. Oral chelation therapy. Consider hospitalization.
≥70	Same as above. Oral chelation therapy and hospitalization. Consult toxicology or a pediatric environmental health specialty team.

Adapted from Centers for Disease Control and Prevention (CDC). Childhood Lead Poisoning Prevention: Recommended Actions Based on Blood Lead Level. Available at: https://www.cdc.gov/nceh/lead/advisory/acclpp/actions-blls.htm. Accessed April 4 2020.

or infectious cause.[41] At the time of initial lead testing, refugees are also screened for anemia and malnutrition.[40]

CLINICS CARE POINTS

- A CBC can reveal important information regarding underlying health conditions, the management of which can improve health outcomes after resettlement.
- Patients with inherited blood cell conditions including thalassemias or hemoglobinopathies are at risk of over iron replacement if not correctly diagnosed.
- Asymptomatic eosinophilia should not be ignored and in this population suggests parasitic infection. If a parasite is found, once treated then a repeat CBC should be performed at least a month later to ensure the eosinophilia is resolving.
- In patients with thrombocytopenia, evaluate for presence and causes of splenomegaly.
- Dental disease should be considered as a potential cause and/or effect of nutritional insufficiency.

- Federal assistance programs, such as Temporary Assistance for Needy Families or Supplemental Nutrition Assistance Program, formally known as the Food Stamp program, are available depending on immigration status.

- Specifically, for refugees from Southeast Asia, screen for betel nut use before starting vitamin D because betel nut may be wrapped in a calcium product.[3,20]

- If possible, work with the resettlement agency or another entity to have language- and culture-appropriate nutrition workshops related to food choices, preparation food labels, and cost on resettlement. It is also important for the refugee clients to be enrolled in the food supplementation programs in which they are eligible.[20]

- Diagnosing asthma with pulmonary function testing is difficult because of language and cultural barriers. To obtain accurate results, interpretation must be provided, and instructions should be clearly described (eg, video).

- All prescribed spacers and nebulizers should have clear instructions (eg, handouts in preferred language with photographs, live demonstration, and teach-back).[42]

- Many refugee patients initially have refugee medical assistance or government insurance but many may have financial constraints in obtaining inhalers. Stepwise therapy and/or formulary inhalers are likely more effective in compliance because of cost.

- There are a multitude of barriers that limit equitable health care access and disproportionally affect vulnerable populations, such as refugees (eg, geographic, transportation, language, sociocultural), and may contribute toward poor understanding of the follow-up recommendations and the need for retesting of blood lead level.

- Low socioeconomic status is a risk factor for EBLL and likely contributes to the prevalence of lead toxicity in refugees.[39]

DISCLOSURE

The authors have nothing to disclose.

REFERENCES

1. Complete blood count with red blood cell indices, white blood cell differential, and platelet count. Centers for Disease Control and Prevention; 2016. Available at: https://www.cdc.gov/immigrantrefugeehealth/guidelines/domestic/general/discussion/complete-blood-count.html. Accessed May 16, 2020.
2. Pottie K, Greenaway C, Feightner J, et al. Evidence-based clinical guidelines for immigrants and refugees including Appendix 15. CMAJ 2011;183(12):E824–925.
3. Walker PF, Barnett ED. Immigrant medicine. 14,21,46. St Louis (MO): Saunders Elsevier; 2007.
4. General and Optional Tests. Centers for Disease Control and Prevention. 2012. Available at: https://www.cdc.gov/immigrantrefugeehealth/guidelines/domestic/general/general-and-optional-tests.html. Accessed May 16, 2020.
5. Clinical Resource For Family Physicians seeing Newly Arrived Refugees and Claimants. RefugeeHealthYYC. Available at: https://www.refugeehealthyyc.ca/for-clinicians. Accessed May 13, 2020.
6. Caring for Kids New to Canada. Canadian Paediatric Society. Available at: https://www.kidsnewtocanada.ca/. Accessed May 13, 2020.
7. Redditt VJ, Graziano D, Janakiram P, et al. Health status of newly arrived refugees in Toronto, Ont: Part 2: chronic diseases. Can Fam Physician 2015 Jul;61(7):e310–5.
8. Zeller M, Verhovsek M. Treating iron deficiency. CMAJ 2017;189(10):E409.

9. PBM. SaskBlood. 2020. Available at: http://saskblood.ca/pbm/. Accessed May 17, 2020.

10. Langan RC. Vitamin B12 deficiency: recognition and management. Am Fam Physician 2017;96(6):384–9.

11. Langan RC, Zawistoski KJ. Update on Vitamin B12 Deficiency. St. Luke's Hospital, Bethlehem, Pennsylvania. Am Fam Physician. 2011 Jun 15;83(12):1425-1430. Available at: https://www.aafp.org/afp/2011/0615/p1425.html. Accessed May 17, 2020.

12. Lanier JB, Park JJ, Callahan RC. Anemia in older adults. Am Fam Physician 2018; 98(7):437-442.

13. Abramson SD, Abramson N. 'Common' uncommon anemias. Am Fam Physician 1999 Feb 15;59(4):851–8.

14. Thalassemias. National Heart Lung and Blood Institute. Available at: https://www. nhlbi.nih.gov/health-topics/thalassemias. Accessed May 16, 2020.

15. Barcellini W, Bianchi P, Fermo E, et al. Hereditary red cell membrane defects: diagnostic and clinical aspects. Blood Transfus 2011;9(3):274–7.

16. Dhaliwal G, Cornett PA, Tierney LM Jr. Hemolytic anemia. Am Fam Physician 2004;69(11):2599–606.

17. Shoenfeld Y, Alkan ML, Asaly A, et al. Benign familial leukopenia and neutropenia in different ethnic groups. Eur J Haematol 1988;41(3):273–7.

18. Available at: https://www.cdc.gov/immigrantrefugeehealth/guidelines/domestic/ intestinal-parasite-flow-chart.html. 2018. Accessed May 12, 2020.

19. Thrombocytopenia: MedlinePlus Medical Encyclopedia. MedlinePlus. Available at: https://medlineplus.gov/ency/article/000586.htm. Accessed May 14, 2020.

20. Sastre L, Haldeman L. Environmental, nutrition and health issues in a US refugee resettlement community. MEDICC Rev 2015;17:18–24.

21. Goel MS, McCarthy EP, Phillips RS, et al. Obesity among US immigrant subgroups by duration of residence. JAMA 2004;292(23):2860–7.

22. McCullough MB, Marks AK. The immigrant paradox and adolescent obesity: examining health behaviors as potential mediators. J Dev Behav Pediatr 2014; 35(2):138–43.

23. Centers for Disease Control and Prevention. Guidelines for the evaluation of the nutritional status and growth in refugee children during the domestic medical screening examination. 2013. Available at: https://www.cdc.gov/ immigrantrefugeehealth/guidelines/domestic/nutrition-growth.html. Accessed May 17, 2020.

24. Sanou D, O'Reilly E, Ngnie-Teta I, et al. Acculturation and nutritional health of immigrants in Canada: a scoping review. J Immigr Minor Health 2014;16(1):24–34.

25. Brown CM, Swaminathan L, Saif NT, et al. Health care for refugee and immigrant adolescents. Prim Care 2020;47(2):291–306.

26. Fabio M. Nutrition for refugee children: risks, screening, and treatment. Curr Probl Pediatr Adolesc Health Care 2014;44(7):188–95.

27. Garcia-Marcos L, Robertson CF, Ross Anderson H, et al, ISAAC Phase Three Study Group. Does migration affect asthma, rhinoconjunctivitis and eczema prevalence? Global findings from the international study of asthma and allergies in childhood. Int J Epidemiol 2014;43(6):1846–54.

28. Cabieses B, Uphoff E, Pinart M, et al. A systematic review on the development of asthma and allergic diseases in relation to international immigration: the leading role of the environment confirmed. PLoS One 2014;9(8):e105347.

29. Yao J, Sbihi H. Prevalence of non-food allergies among non-immigrants, long-time immigrants and recent immigrants in Canada. Can J Public Health 2016; 107(4–5):e461–6.
30. Silverberg JI, Simpson EL, Durkin HG, et al. Prevalence of allergic disease in foreign-born American children. JAMA Pediatr 2013;167(6):554–60.
31. Holguin F, Moughrabieh MA, Ojeda V, et al. Respiratory health in migrant populations: a crisis overlooked. Ann Am Thorac Soc 2017;14(2):153–9.
32. Annamalai A, editor. Refugee health care: an essential medical guide. New York: Springer Science & Business Media; 2014.
33. Lidsky TI, Schneider JS. Lead neurotoxicity in children: basic mechanisms and clinical correlates. Brain 2003;126(1):5–19.
34. Bellinger DC. Very low lead exposures and children's neurodevelopment. Curr Opin Pediatr 2008;20(2):172–7.
35. Centers for Disease Control and Prevention. Low level head exposure harms children: a renewed call for primary prevention: Report of the Advisory Committee on Childhood Lead Poisoning Prevention of the Centers for Disease Control and Prevention". 2012; 1–65.
36. Centers for Disease Control and Prevention. Blood lead levels in children aged 1–5 years—United States, 1999–2010. MMWR 2013;62(13):245–8.
37. World Health Organization. Childhood lead poisoning 2010. p. 1–69. Available at: http://www.who.int/ceh/publications/leadguidance.pdf. Accessed July 23, 2018.
38. Centers for Disease Control and Prevention. Lead poisoning prevention in newly arrived refugee children: tool kit. 2016.
39. Binns HJ, Kim D, Campbell C. Targeted screening for elevated blood lead levels: populations at high risk. Pediatrics 2001;108:1364–6.
40. Childhood Lead Poisoning Prevention. Available at: https://www.cdc.gov/nceh/lead/prevention/refugees.htm. Accessed April 4, 2020.
41. Richardson M. Microcytic anemia. Pediatr Rev 2007;28(1):5–14.
42. Pollart SM, Elward KS. Overview of changes to asthma guidelines: diagnosis and screening. Am Fam Physician 2009;79(9):761–7.

Preventive Care and Management of Chronic Diseases in Immigrant Adults

Colleen Payton, PhD, MPH[a],*, Sarah Kimball, MD[b,c],
Nicole Chow Ahrenholz, MD[d,e], Mark L. Wieland, MD, MPH[f]

KEYWORDS

- Chronic disease management • Preventive care • Immigrants
- Cardiovascular disease • Diabetes • Cancer • Immunizations

KEY POINTS

- Immigrants are a heterogeneous population with between-group and within-group differences in chronic disease risk factors.
- Immigrants generally have healthier chronic disease risk profiles compared with the US population, but risk increases with time in the United States.
- Chronic disease management may be an unfamiliar concept because of minimal preventive care and limited access to acute care in immigrants' countries of origin.
- Health care providers should prioritize chronic disease screening and follow up regularly to encourage preventive care and self-management of chronic disease.

INTRODUCTION

The countries with the highest proportion of foreign-born people living in the United States include Mexico, China, India, Philippines, El Salvador, Vietnam, Cuba, Dominican Republic, Korea, and Guatemala.[1] Immigrants are a heterogeneous population with between-group and within-group differences in chronic disease prevalence. Some chronic disease risk factors are lower in countries from which immigrants are migrating compared with the United States, including alcohol consumption, obesity, and increased cholesterol level.[2] Other risk factors are higher, including high blood

a School of Nursing and Public Health, Moravian College, 1200 Main Street, Bethlehem, PA 18018, USA; b Immigrant & Refugee Health Center, Boston Medical Center, 725 Albany Street, 43 Suite 5b, Boston, MA 02118, USA; c Boston University School of Medicine, 72 E Concord St, Boston, MA 02118, USA; d International Medicine Clinic, Harborview Medical Center, 325 9th Avenue Box 359895, Seattle, WA 98104, USA; e University of Washington School of Medicine, 1959 NE Pacific St, Seattle, WA 98195, USA; f Community Internal Medicine, Mayo Clinic, 200 First Street Southwest, Rochester, MN 55905, USA
* Corresponding author.
E-mail address: PaytonC@moravian.edu

Prim Care Clin Office Pract 48 (2021) 83–97
https://doi.org/10.1016/j.pop.2020.09.006
0095-4543/21/© 2020 Elsevier Inc. All rights reserved.

primarycare.theclinics.com

pressure, increased fasting blood glucose level, and smoking tobacco. Chronic disease prevalence is generally lower in countries from which immigrants are migrating compared with the United States.[3] The cause-specific mortality is higher for diabetes mellitus and stroke compared with the United States (**Fig. 1**). In this article, chronic disease prevalence, prevention, and disease management among immigrants to the United States are examined. Clinical pearls, pitfalls, and case examples are constructed to show the complexity and prioritization of care.

CHRONIC DISEASE PREVALENCE, PREVENTION, AND MANAGEMENT
Cardiovascular Disease and Associated Risk Factors

Immigrants generally have healthier cardiovascular risk profiles compared with the US population, including lower risk of cardiovascular death.[4] Cardiovascular risk factors tend to increase with time in the United States, including obesity,[5] hyperlipidemia,[6] hypertension,[7] and diabetes mellitus,[8] as does known cardiovascular disease.[9] There are significant differences in cardiovascular disease outcomes depending on country of origin and host country. For example, cardiovascular risk is high among South Asian immigrants on arrival, and remains high with sustained residency.[10]

Clinicians are important cardiovascular disease advocates. Clinicians can embrace the differences in risk factors between and within immigrant groups to tailor a treatment and prevention plan. Newly arrived immigrants with low cardiovascular risk

	Alcohol use disorders	Cardiovascular disease	Chronic kidney disease	Chronic respiratory disease	Diabetes mellitus	Neoplasms	Non-communicable diseases	Stroke	Substance use disorders
United States	4.30	277.76	26.15	60.64	21.11	215.30	779.99	53.05	25.12
Mexico	3.91	127.82	51.38	27.11	50.62	76.86	442.48	28.96	4.98
China	1.49	309.95	12.45	71.48	10.85	184.56	662.16	149.37	3.08
India	2.09	190.70	16.21	92.11	18.44	67.33	455.60	52.60	2.90
Philippines	1.38	210.26	32.91	31.95	25.17	76.62	446.68	70.84	1.95
El Salvador	15.53	161.74	67.47	21.90	35.33	92.62	497.01	33.17	16.55
Vietnam	1.08	209.21	18.08	37.39	24.38	125.46	498.17	116.12	2.38
Cuba	6.18	330.49	20.57	38.73	15.55	230.32	762.60	86.78	6.86
Dominican Republic	1.56	229.46	22.09	16.32	22.84	95.17	461.30	67.33	2.72
Korea	1.95	126.80	11.57	26.53	22.25	175.71	473.50	58.21	2.26
Guatemala	9.98	88.68	29.93	11.79	32.68	65.19	317.51	25.85	12.09

Fig. 1. Cause-specific mortality per 100,000 by countries with the largest proportion of immigrants to the United States, 2017. Korea reported using South Korea data. Color coding: green, less than United States value; red, greater than United States value. (*Data from* United States Census Bureau. Place of birth for the foreign-born population in the United States. Available at: https://data.census.gov/cedsci/table?tid=ACSDT1Y2016.B05006&q= B05006. Accessed April 16 2020; and Global Health Data Exchange. GBD Results Tool. Available at: http://ghdx.healthdata.org/gbd-results-tool. Accessed April 16 2020.)

face disproportionate barriers to sustaining their health. Proactive counseling and periodic follow-up are important for diet, physical activity, and other health-promoting behaviors. Clinicians can advocate tailored interventions to address unique risk factors and to attenuate the accumulation of cardiovascular risk.[11] Evidence-based health promotion programs such as diabetes prevention interventions may be tailored and led by members of specific immigrant communities.[12]

Diet and physical activity

Cardiovascular risk factors among many immigrant groups are mediated by physical activity and diet. Immigrants often have lower physical activity and eat a less healthy diet after arrival.[13,14] Environmental factors include lifestyle transitions that require less physical activity, disproportionately low access to safe spaces for physical activity, and an obesogenic food environment compounded by increased risk for food insecurity. Social factors include low socioeconomic position and cultural considerations such as identity threat and a lack of norms around leisure-time physical activity.[15,16] Acculturation was associated with lower dietary quality but higher leisure-time physical activity.[17,18]

Obesity

Overweight and obesity prevalence is higher among immigrants from Mexico, Central America, and the Caribbean.[19] Obesity rates generally increase after arrival; children of immigrants have an increased risk for obesity and its associated complications. Successful obesity prevention interventions should be initiated within 15 years after arrival.[5]

Hypertension

Hypertension is the most important modifiable risk factor for cardiovascular disease, and it disproportionately affects immigrant populations. There is significant heterogeneity of prevalence, with high rates among immigrants from Southeast Asia, Mexico, Central America, Africa, and the Caribbean.[20] Immigrants with hypertension are more likely to have poorly controlled disease than native-born patients.[21]

Diabetes

Immigrants have a higher diabetes prevalence compared with host countries and tend to develop diabetes at a younger age.[22] Immigrants from South Asia, Latin America and the Caribbean, Central America, sub-Saharan Africa, and the Indian subcontinent had a higher prevalence compared with western Europe and North America.[8,23] Risk factors for immigrants include female gender, lower socioeconomic status, lower education levels, longer time after arrival, public or no health insurance, lack of usual source of care, and low neighborhood walkability.[8,23–25]

Diabetes screening should start soon after resettlement.[23] Diabetes screening increased with the number of primary care physician visits, indicating that routine visits lead to opportunistic care.[26] Screening rates were higher for immigrants from South Asia, the Caribbean, Mexico, and Latin America compared with Europe, Central Asia, and the United States.[26] Neighborhoods with low income and high immigration levels had lower rates of glucose and cholesterol screenings compared with neighborhoods with higher income and lower immigration levels.[27] Multiphasic screening, 2 or more screening tests combined and offered to a large population, could increase chronic disease screening.[27]

Immigrants had higher hemoglobin A1c (HbA1c) levels and lower odds of treating diabetes with insulin,[22,28] although there is heterogeneity in diabetes-related mortality.[4,22] Providers should have familiarity with a community's traditional dietary practices when counseling about diabetes management. Immigrants may have cultural beliefs about insulin, which could affect self-monitoring and medication adherence. Those of Hispanic or Asian descent may fear injections; they may also perceive insulin as a failure to self-manage diabetes and the reason for other complications.[29] Access to insulin and related supplies varies based on insurance.

Chronic Kidney Disease

Approximately 0.3% of 444,356 recently resettled adult refugees were diagnosed with chronic kidney disease (CKD); there was a correlation between CKD and tuberculosis, obesity, diabetes, hypertension, and tobacco use.[30] There was a correlation between discrimination and CKD among Caribbean black people born in the United States but not among recent (<5 years) immigrants.[30,31]

CKD management is important to slow the progression of kidney damage. CKD care is not as accessible or affordable in low-income and middle-income countries, which have a lower prevalence of publicly funded kidney replacement therapy, including hemodialysis, peritoneal dialysis, and kidney transplant.[32] Many regions have a nephrologist shortage, including Africa, the Middle East, South Asia, and Oceania and Southeast Asia.[32]

CKD management is difficult for undocumented immigrants with end-stage renal disease. In one study, undocumented immigrants had access to emergency dialysis, but only half had access to maintenance dialysis, which was more accessible in states with a higher prevalence of undocumented immigrants.[33] Undocumented immigrants on dialysis had a lower coronary artery disease and diabetes incidence compared US residents; potential kidney donors were available for most.[34] Transplants would be a cost-savings societal solution because 35% of nephrologists report uncompensated dialysis care for undocumented immigrants with end-stage renal disease.[33,34]

Chronic Obstructive Pulmonary Disease

Immigrants have a lower chronic obstructive pulmonary disease (COPD) prevalence and related mortality than US-born populations.[35] Primary risk factors include exposure to tobacco smoke, occupational exposure, and indoor and outdoor air pollution, including cooking smoke. Cultural and language differences affect patients' understanding and disease management, which can lead to barriers to care.[36] COPD requires education, self-management, and long-term medication use to prevent complications and reduce morbidity. Most COPD medications are delivered via devices (metered-dose inhalers, dry-powder inhalers, and nebulizers) that require proper technique and dexterity; many patients require more than 1 medication. Insurance formularies change frequently; a patient might have to switch to a different device, causing confusion. Busy dispensing pharmacies often lack the time and resources to thoroughly educate patients with limited English proficiency on proper technique. Regular appointments with a multidisciplinary care team provide ongoing education and improve adherence.

Cancer

Cancer-related morbidity and mortality are generally lower for immigrants than native-born populations in high-income countries. Incidences of cancers associated with lifestyle norms are generally lower, including colorectal, lung, breast, ovarian, prostate, and pancreatic cancer. Cancer incidence associated with infectious diseases are often higher among immigrant groups, including Kaposi sarcoma and gastric, liver, and cervical cancer.[4,37]

Cancer risk increases with duration in the United States. Immigrants receive fewer recommended preventive cancer screenings, which can cause late-stage diagnosis and higher disease-related mortality.[38,39] Reasons for lower screening include individuals' knowledge, beliefs, language proficiency, access to care, insurance status, institutional practices, and health care provider characteristics or competencies.[40–43] Peer navigators have improved cancer screening rates for immigrants.[44]

Substance Use Disorders

Substance use disorder (SUD) prevalence is lower among immigrants than US-born populations. Immigrants were less likely to meet criteria for alcohol, marijuana, cocaine, and opioid use disorders compared with US-born individuals (adjusted odds ratio [AOR] = 0.50, 95% confidence interval [CI] = 0.43–0.58) or lifetime SUD (AOR = 0.38, 95% CI = 0.34–0.43).[45] Cultural norms in many regions strongly discourage substance use compared with Western culture. Immigrants may experience real or perceived vulnerability in society and fear the risk of criminal justice system consequences, such as denied admission, deportation, or denied citizenship.[46]

SUD risk factors should alert clinicians to investigate further and screening should continue over time. Alcohol use disorder rates tend to increase over time in the United States. SUD rates generally increase with immigrant generation, longer time in the United States, and lower age at arrival, which are all surrogates for acculturation to Western norms.[47] Socioeconomic stressors can lead to increased SUD risk, including discrimination, marginalization, disruption of social ties, unemployment, substandard housing/homelessness, and stressors caused by immigration status.[48] Few culturally appropriate, trauma-informed models have been studied to evaluate the best approaches to supporting recovery.

Tobacco and Betel Nut

Tobacco consumption rates vary dramatically worldwide. US immigrants have variable exposure to tobacco products and often have limited access to cessation tools. The World Health Organization projected that the global number of men using tobacco was declining, and that an increasing number of countries have tobacco cessation support measures.[49] Electronic nicotine delivery systems (electronic cigarettes or vapes) are increasingly available, and their health consequences are relatively unstudied. Clinicians should cast an inquisitive and broad net when asking about prior tobacco exposure and treatment access.

Betel nut is harvested from the *Areca* palm and is consumed broadly throughout the world. It is sold in many forms, often wrapped into a betel quid or paan. Betel nut contains a variety of potentially carcinogenic objects, which are generally chewed and placed in the mouth between the lips and gum. Regular exposure can cause red-stained teeth and lips and has been associated with higher rates of lip, mouth, tongue, throat, and esophageal cancer.[50]

Adult Immunizations

Immunizations are a cornerstone of preventive health care, but disparities exist in rates between foreign-born and US-born populations.[51] One study showed lower immunization rates in Russian and Ukrainian communities and higher rates in Mexican and Indian communities in Washington.[52] Disparities exist because of cultural factors, knowledge barriers, insufficient access to health care, and vaccine hesitancy.[53]

Certain incentives exist to encourage immunizations in newly arrived immigrants. Age-appropriate immunizations are required for refugees to adjust their status to lawful permanent residents (getting a green card), an important step in qualifying for certain

Table 1		
Approach to immunization of adult immigrants without records		
Vaccines	Required for Adults (≥18 y Old) Seeking Lawful Permanent Resident Status	Approach for Adults Who Have no Records
Hepatitis A	No	Recommended if risk factors for HAV infection or severe disease from HAV
Hepatitis B	No	Check serology and recommended immunization for at-risk individuals. Hepatitis B serologies should not be sent within 30 d of suspected vaccination
Hib	No	Age-appropriate immunization per ACIP recommendations
HPV	No	Recommended age-appropriate immunization per ACIP recommendations
Influenza	Yes (required during flu season, October 1–March 31)	1 dose recommended annually
Meningococcus	No	Age-appropriate immunization per ACIP recommendations
MMR	Yes, if born in 1957 or later	Immunize if born after 1957
Pneumococcus	Yes, if ≥65 y old or risk factors	Age-appropriate immunization
Polio	No	Vaccination not needed unless planning travel to endemic area (CDC)
Td/Tdap	Yes (substitute 1-time dose of Tdap for Td booster; then boost with Td every 10 y)	Age-appropriate immunization per ACIP recommendations
Varicella (chickenpox)	Yes	Check serology and immunize if naive
Zoster (shingles)	No	Recommended age-appropriate immunization per ACIP recommendations

Abbreviations: ACIP, Advisory Committee on Immunization Practices; CDC, US Centers for Disease Control and Prevention; HAV, hepatitis A virus; Hib, *Haemophilus influenzae* type b; HPV, human papilloma virus; MMR, measles, mumps, and rubella; Td, Tdap, tetanus and diphtheria; tetanus, diphtheria, and pertussis.
   Data from Refs.[56,74,75]

benefits and a requirement toward citizenship.[54] Some immunizations are required for enrollment in school and work. Many immigrants arrive with limited documentation of prior immunizations.[55] Clinicians have to make decisions to empirically vaccinate, check serologies for immunity, or combine both approaches (**Table 1**). Immunizations administered outside the United States that are compatible with Advisory Committee on Immunization Practices recommendations should be considered valid.[56]

Dental, Vision, and Hearing Care

If dental, vision, and hearing care is not addressed, it can lead to poor health outcomes, such as diabetes, cardiovascular disease, depression, falls, and hospitalizations.[57]

Many immigrants have poor access to these services before US arrival and limited access after migration. Clinicians have a low participation in Medicaid depending on the state; access to care is often through community health centers, which have limited capacity.[58] Traditional Medicare has limited vision coverage and does not cover dental or hearing care.[57] Many adults have to pay out of pocket for these services, resulting in a high need and low use.[57]

Dental care

There is limited research on dental health for adult immigrants. Chinese and Hispanic older adult immigrants were less likely to visit the dentist, more likely to have lost a tooth because of disease, and more likely to experience lower satisfaction when visiting the dentist compared with white patients.[59] Dental visit predictors included speaking English for older adult immigrants from China and education level for Hispanic patients.[59] Dental visit facilitators among immigrants include patients reporting having a dentist to visit if needed, current dental health problems, having a primary care provider, and dental insurance.[60] Dental care barriers for immigrants include transportation costs, fear, and lack of preventive care focus.[60] Systems-level barriers include the lack of diversity in the dental profession, the need for interpretation services, insufficient access to professional interpreters, and the need for more training and education on diverse cultures.[58,61–63] Previous research showed that dental hygiene students underestimated potential barriers and not all patient needs were addressed during the initial visit.[63]

Vision care

The National Health and Nutrition Examination Survey (2003–2008) showed differences in visual acuity between immigrants and US citizens.[64] US citizens had a higher prevalence of myopia.[64] Naturalized citizens and noncitizens had lower visual acuity, were less likely to wear glasses, and had a higher prevalence of legal blindness.[64] Naturalized citizens had significantly higher prevalence of hyperopia, diabetes, and surgery for myopia compared with US citizens.[64] Vision care can improve quality of life because it allows people to work, drive, and complete daily activities.[65] Immigrant populations are in need of access to prescription eyeglasses and contact lenses.[65] Vision stations include tables for eye testing and adjustable glasses fitting at health outreach events; they are a feasible, low-cost method for corrective vision needs, including adjustable glasses, ordering custom lenses, and referrals for eye concerns.[65] Vision screening at health fairs can occur without cost or the need for insurance.[64]

Hearing care

Hearing loss among US children is 7.5% higher when including immigrant children from Mexico and China, suggesting higher rates of hearing loss in immigrant children.[66] Chronic otitis media is more common in developing countries and is associated with hearing loss.[67] Agriculture, forestry, fishing, and hunting workers experience high noise levels, which can lead to occupational hearing loss; approximately 37% of these workers are immigrants.[68,69] A higher proportion of immigrants work in jobs with high noise levels and may not request hearing protection from their employer because of fear of deportation.[68–70] Hearing impairment risk is higher among immigrants with limited English proficiency.[68–70] Low acculturation and low personal attenuation rating (hearing protection fit testing) were associated in a study of mostly Hispanic immigrants exposed to noise at work.[71] Immigrant farm workers inconsistently used hearing protection and had a low-risk perception of job-related injury.[72] Hearing-related job training was reported less frequently among workers with limited

English proficiency.[72] Workplaces should regularly communicate hearing protection information and conduct safety audits in workers' preferred languages with cultural sensitivity.[71]

CLINICAL CASE STUDIES
Chronic Disease and Prevention Case Study

G.S., a 50-year-old recent immigrant from Guatemala, presents for a work-related injury; it is his first interaction with health care in the United States. His blood pressure is 168/98 mm Hg. He is due for colorectal cancer screening. He is reluctant to take hypertension medications or screen for cancer because he has no symptoms and thinks cancer screening could be dangerous. Telephonic interpretation is challenging because of differences in dialect. The patient does not have insurance and worries about the cost.

Plan

Schedule a hypertension education visit with a clinician and an in-person professional medical interpreter. Recheck his blood pressure after his injury resolves. Arrange frequent follow-up until adherence is sustained and trust is established. Assign a peer navigator (community health worker or promotora) for cancer screening navigation, while implementing regional, no-cost screening options for uninsured patients.

Initial Screening Case Study

F.M., a 49-year-old refugee from Somalia, presents to establish care. She has no known past medical history and minimal access to health care before US arrival 2 months ago. She expresses hesitation about invasive tests and exercising in her neighborhood or a traditional gym. Her vitals are unremarkable except for a body mass index of 32.

Plan

Review overseas results and immunizations before ordering additional tests. Order routine immigrant screening laboratory tests, HbA1c, lipid panel, and chemistry panel including renal function. Initiate the tetanus and measles, mumps and rubella (MMR) series, and plan to give hepatitis A and B immunizations if indicated based on prior tests and laboratory evaluation. Refer her to a nutritionist who has familiarity with a traditional Somali diet and connections with community programs providing fresh fruits and vegetables to low-income individuals. Provide counseling on exercise programs such as the women-only swim program offered at the community pool. Schedule her for close follow-up to discuss laboratory results and continue the immunization series. Defer cancer screening discussions until a rapport is built and she gains familiarity with the medical system.

Immunization Case Study

Y.B., a 58-year-old recently arrived Ukrainian refugee, presents to establish care with no overseas medical records. She is found to be immune to hepatitis A and varicella during the domestic medical examination, a refugee health screening. Her hepatitis B serologies and antigen are negative. She declines immunizations because she believes they are dangerous. She plans to start working as a nursing assistant.

Plan

Acknowledge her hesitancy, provide education about vaccine safety, and inform her about the immunizations required for adjustment of status and work in health care.

Table 2
Clinical pearls and pitfalls related to chronic disease management and prevention for immigrants to the United States

Chronic Conditions	Clinical Pearls	Clinical Pitfalls
Chronic conditions in general	• Premigration access to chronic disease screening and treatment varies by country of origin • Chronic disease risk factors can be from premigration or postmigration exposure, treatment, or barriers to care • Long-term counseling is critical to prevent adoption of unhealthy risk behaviors because immigrants tend to accumulate behaviors of the US population. • Clinicians should take a holistic approach to patient care that accounts for the social determinants of health because chronic disease risk factors frequently overlap with socioeconomic risk factors	• United States Preventive Services Task Force guidelines need to be adapted because they are contingent on appropriate prior screening and were developed based on US population prevalence • Trained medical interpretation is critical for communication about chronic diseases with immigrants who have limited English proficiency • Some immigrants lack insurance coverage for chronic disease screening and care because of their immigration status • Chronic disease management may be an unfamiliar concept because of minimal preventive care and limited access to acute care in the country of origin
Cardiovascular disease	• Cardiovascular risk factors are often lower than in the general population immediately after immigration, including physical inactivity, unhealthy diet, tobacco use, hypertension, hyperlipidemia, obesity, and diabetes • Accumulation of cardiovascular risk factors occurs disproportionately after immigration • Interventions to reduce cardiovascular risk should start soon after arrival and continue as part of preventive care in order to have maximal impact	• There is heterogeneity in cardiovascular disease prevalence and risk factors depending on country of origin and socioeconomic status
Hypertension	• Hypertension disproportionately affects immigrant populations; immigrants are less likely to achieve blood pressure control than US-born patients	• Patients without preventive care experience may struggle with treatment adherence related to asymptomatic conditions such as hypertension
Diabetes	• Many faiths recommend periods of religious fasting, which may require adjustments to the timing of diabetes medications to avoid hypoglycemia	• Immigrants may have cultural beliefs about insulin, which could affect self-monitoring and medication adherence • Access to insulin and related supplies may be limited by health insurance coverage

(continued on next page)

Table 2 (continued)		
Chronic Conditions	Clinical Pearls	Clinical Pitfalls
CKD	• Treatment of CKD before end-stage renal disease is frequently inaccessible or unaffordable in countries of origin for immigrants; this is partially caused by a global shortage of nephrologists and related services	• Access to dialysis is often limited for individuals with insecure immigration statuses in the United States
COPD	• There are high rates of exposure to air pollution, indoor cooking smoke, and occupational dust and chemicals internationally compared with the United States; clinicians should screen for these risk factors	• COPD medication devices and regimens can be confusing, particularly for patients with low English proficiency
Cancer	• Cancer incidence associated with infectious diseases are higher among immigrant groups. Cancers associated with lifestyle factors are lower among immigrant groups • Age-adjusted cancer risk increases with time lived in the United States	• Cancer screening is generally lower in immigrant groups • Barriers to cancer screening include knowledge, beliefs, language proficiency, access to care, and institutional practices
SUD	• Many treatment programs and modalities are not accessible for individuals with a vulnerable immigration status	• Immigrants may under-report substance use out of concern for stigma and implications for future immigration options
Tobacco and betel nut	• Clinicians should inquire about smoking, betel nut, and electronic nicotine delivery system use	• Few SUD and tobacco treatment programs are equipped to take into account cultural variations in use and treatment
Immunizations	• Age-appropriate immunizations are required for adjustment of status (ie, green card) application	• Many immigrants arrive with missing or incomplete immunization records
Dental, vision, and hearing care	• The prevalence of visual acuity diagnoses and legal blindness is higher among immigrant groups • Immigrants are less likely to wear glasses • Hearing impairment risk is higher among immigrants with limited English proficiency	• Many medical insurances have limited vision, dental, and hearing coverage, resulting in patients having to pay out of pocket for these services • Access to care is often through community health centers, which may have limited capacity

Encourage her to start her vaccination series for hepatitis B, tetanus, and MMR (needed because she was born after 1957). She has no indications for vaccines for polio, *Haemophilus influenzae* type b, meningococcus, varicella-zoster virus, or pneumococcus.

Pearls and Pitfalls

Primary care providers identified chronic conditions among the high-priority conditions for recently arriving immigrants, including diabetes mellitus, dental caries and periodontal disease, cancer of the cervix, and vision screening.[73] Clinical pearls and pitfalls were constructed to show the complexity and prioritization of care (**Table 2**).

CLINICS CARE POINTS

- Immigrants may have variable access to chronic disease screening and treatment in their countries of origin and host country, often limited by their immigration status.
- Immigrants face barriers to chronic disease management and preventive care, including health insurance access, linguistic challenges, lack of culturally sensitive care, limited records, and acculturation.
- Health care providers should prioritize chronic disease screening and follow up regularly to encourage preventive care and self-management of chronic disease.

DISCLOSURE

The authors have nothing to disclose.

REFERENCES

1. Place of birth for the foreign-born population in the United States. United States Census Bureau. Available at: https://data.census.gov/cedsci/table?tid=ACSDT1Y2016.B05006&q=B05006. Accessed April 16, 2020.
2. Noncommunicable diseases risk factors. World Health Organization. Available at: https://www.who.int/data/gho/data/themes/topics/topic-details/GHO/noncommunicable-diseases—risk-factors. Accessed April 16, 2020.
3. GBD Results Tool. Global Health Data Exchange. Available at: http://ghdx.healthdata.org/gbd-results-tool. Accessed April 16, 2020.
4. Singh GK, Siahpush M. All-cause and cause-specific mortality of immigrants and native born in the United States. Am J Public Health 2001;91(3):392–9.
5. Goel MS, McCarthy EP, Phillips RS, et al. Obesity among US immigrant subgroups by duration of residence. JAMA 2004;292(23):2860–7.
6. Koya DL, Egede LE. Association between length of residence and cardiovascular disease risk factors among an ethnically diverse group of United States immigrants. J Gen Intern Med 2007;22(6):841–6.
7. Steffen PR, Smith TB, Larson M, et al. Acculturation to Western society as a risk factor for high blood pressure: a meta-analytic review. Psychosom Med 2006; 68(3):386–97.
8. Creatore MI, Moineddin R, Booth G, et al. Age- and sex-related prevalence of diabetes mellitus among immigrants to Ontario, Canada. CMAJ 2010;182(8):781–9.
9. Lutsey PL, Diez Roux AV, Jacobs DR Jr, et al. Associations of acculturation and socioeconomic status with subclinical cardiovascular disease in the multi-ethnic study of atherosclerosis. Am J Public Health 2008;98(11):1963–70.
10. Sohail QZ, Chu A, Rezai MR, et al. The risk of ischemic heart disease and stroke among immigrant populations: a systematic review. Can J Cardiol 2015;31(9): 1160–8.
11. Renzaho AMN, Mellor D, Boulton K, et al. Effectiveness of prevention programmes for obesity and chronic diseases among immigrants to developed countries - a systematic review. Public Health Nutr 2010;13(3):438–50.

12. Lagisetty PA, Priyadarshini S, Terrell S, et al. Culturally targeted strategies for diabetes prevention in minority population. Diabetes Edu 2017;43(1):54–77.

13. Centers for Disease Control and Prevention (CDC). Prevalence of fruit and vegetable consumption and physical activity by race/ethnicity–United States, 2005. MMWR Morb Mortal Wkly Rep 2007;56(13):301–4.

14. Crespo CJ, Smit E, Andersen RE, et al. Race/ethnicity, social class and their relation to physical inactivity during leisure time: results from the Third National Health and Nutrition Examination Survey, 1988–1994. Am J Prev Med 2000;18(1):46–53.

15. Dunn JR, Dyck I. Social determinants of health in Canada's immigrant population: results from the National Population Health Survey. Social Sci Med 2000;51(11): 1573–93.

16. Caperchione CM, Kolt GS, Mummery WK. Physical activity in culturally and linguistically diverse migrant groups to Western society: a review of barriers, enablers and experiences. Sports Med 2009;39(3):167–77.

17. Gerber M, Barker D, Pühse U. Acculturation and physical activity among immigrants: a systematic review. J Public Health 2012;20(3):313–41.

18. Abraído-Lanza AF, Chao MT, Flórez KR. Do healthy behaviors decline with greater acculturation? Implications for the Latino mortality paradox. Soc Sci Med 2005; 61(6):1243–55.

19. Oza-Frank R, Narayan KMV. Overweight and diabetes prevalence among US immigrants. Am J Public Health 2010;100(4):661–8.

20. Commodore-Mensah Y, Selvin E, Aboagye J, et al. Hypertension, overweight/obesity, and diabetes among immigrants in the United States: an analysis of the 2010-2016 National Health Interview Survey. BMC Public Health 2018; 18(1):773.

21. Agyemang C, Kieft S, Snijder MB, et al. Hypertension control in a large multi-ethnic cohort in Amsterdam, The Netherlands: the HELIUS study. Int J Cardiol 2015;183:180–9.

22. Agyemang C, van den Born B-J. Non-communicable diseases in migrants: an expert review. J Trav Med 2019;26(2). https://doi.org/10.1093/jtm/tay107.

23. Oza-Frank R, Stephenson R, Narayan KMV. Diabetes prevalence by length of residence among US immigrants. J Immigr Minor Health 2011;13(1):1–8.

24. Dallo FJ, Wilson FA, Stimpson JP. Quality of diabetes care for immigrants in the U.S. Diabetes Care 2009;32(8):1459–63.

25. Booth GL, Creatore MI, Moineddin R, et al. Unwalkable neighborhoods, poverty, and the risk of diabetes among recent immigrants to Canada compared with long-term residents. Diabetes Care 2013;36(2):302–8.

26. Creatore MI, Booth GL, Manuel DG, et al. Diabetes screening among immigrants: a population-based urban cohort study. Diabetes Care 2012;35(4):754–61.

27. Borkhoff CM, Saskin R, Rabeneck L, et al. Disparities in receipt of screening tests for cancer, diabetes and high cholesterol in Ontario, Canada: a population-based study using area-based methods. Can J Public Health 2013;104(4):e284–90.

28. Hsueh L, Vrany EA, Patel JS, et al. Associations between immigrant status and pharmacological treatments for diabetes in U.S. adults. Health Psychol 2018; 37(1):61–9.

29. Rebolledo JA, Arellano R. Cultural differences and considerations when initiating insulin. Diabetes Spectr 2016;29(3):185–90.

30. Bardenheier BH, Pavkov ME, Winston CA, et al. Prevalence of tuberculosis disease among adult US-bound refugees with chronic kidney disease. J Immigr Minor Health 2019;21(6):1275–81.

31. Nguyen AW, Hamler TC, Cobb RJ. Discrimination and chronic kidney disease among Caribbean blacks: the effects of immigration and social status. Race Soc Probl 2018;10(3):248–58.
32. Bello AK, Levin A, Tonelli M, et al. Assessment of global kidney health care status. JAMA 2017;317(18):1864–81.
33. Hurley L, Kempe A, Crane LA, et al. Care of undocumented individuals with ESRD: a national survey of US nephrologists. Am J Kidney Dis 2009;53(6):940–9.
34. Linden EA, Cano J, Coritsidis GN. Kidney transplantation in undocumented immigrants with ESRD: a policy whose time has come? Am J Kidney Dis 2012;60(3): 354–9.
35. Singh GK, Hiatt RA. Trends and disparities in socioeconomic and behavioural characteristics, life expectancy, and cause-specific mortality of native-born and foreign-born populations in the United States, 1979-2003. Int J Epidemiol 2006; 35(4):903–19.
36. Shahin W, Stupans I, Kennedy G. Health beliefs and chronic illnesses of refugees: a systematic review. Ethn Health 2018;11:1–13.
37. Arnold M, Razum O, Coebergh J-W. Cancer risk diversity in non-western migrants to Europe: An overview of the literature. Eur J Cancer 2010;46(14):2647–59.
38. Jacobs EA, Karavolos K, Rathouz PJ, et al. Limited English proficiency and breast and cervical cancer screening in a multiethnic population. Am J Public Health 2005;95(8):1410–6.
39. Li CI, Malone KE, Daling JR. Differences in breast cancer stage, treatment, and survival by race and ethnicity. Arch Intern Med 2003;163(1):49–56.
40. Adunlin G, Cyrus JW, Asare M, et al. Barriers and facilitators to breast and cervical cancer screening among immigrants in the United States. J Immigr Minor Health 2019;21(3):606–58.
41. Tran MT, Jeong MB, Nguyen VV, et al. Colorectal cancer beliefs, knowledge, and screening among Filipino, Hmong, and Korean Americans. Cancer 2018; 124(Suppl 7):1552–9.
42. Nápoles AM, Santoyo-Olsson J, Stewart AL, et al. Physician counseling on colorectal cancer screening and receipt of screening among Latino patients. J Gen Intern Med 2015;30(4):483–9.
43. Green AR, Peters-Lewis A, Percac-Lima S, et al. Barriers to screening colonoscopy for low-income Latino and white patients in an urban community health center. J Gen Intern Med 2008;23(6):834–40.
44. Genoff MC, Zaballa A, Gany F, et al. Navigating language barriers: a systematic review of patient navigators' impact on cancer screening for limited English proficient patients. J Gen Intern Med 2016;31(4):426–34.
45. Salas-Wright CP, Vaughn MG, Clark Goings TT, et al. Substance use disorders among immigrants in the United States: A research update. Addict Behav 2018;76:169–73.
46. Vaughn MG, Salas-Wright CP, DeLisi M, et al. The immigrant paradox: immigrants are less antisocial than native-born Americans. Soc Psychiatry Psychiatr Epidemiol 2014;49(7):1129–37.
47. Horyniak D, Melo JS, Farrell RM, et al. Epidemiology of substance use among forced migrants: a global systematic review. PLoS One 2016;11(7):e0159134.
48. Melo JS, Mittal ML, Horyniak D, et al. Injection drug use trajectories among migrant populations: a narrative review. Subst Use Misuse 2018;53(9):1558–70.
49. World Health Organization. WHO report on the global tobacco epidemic, 2008: the MPOWER package. Geneva, Switzerland: World Health Organization; 2008. Available at: https://www.who.int/tobacco/mpower/2009/gtcr_download/en/.

50. IARC Working Group on the Evaluation of Carcinogenic Risks to Humans. Betel-quid and areca-nut chewing and some areca-nut derived nitrosamines. IARC Monogr Eval Carcinog Risks Hum 2004;85:1–334.

51. Lu P-J, Rodriguez-Lainz A, O'Halloran A, et al. Adult vaccination disparities among foreign-born populations in the U.S., 2012. Am J Prev Med 2014;47(6): 722–33.

52. Wolf E, Rowhani-Rahbar A, Tasslimi A, et al. Parental country of birth and child-hood vaccination uptake in Washington State. Pediatrics 2016;138(1). https://doi.org/10.1542/peds.2015-4544.

53. Wilson L, Rubens-Augustson T, Murphy M, et al. Barriers to immunization among newcomers: a systematic review. Vaccine 2018;36(8):1055–62.

54. Vaccination Requirements. USCIS. 2020. Available at: https://www.uscis.gov/tools/designated-civil-surgeons/vaccination-requirements. [Accessed 17 April 2020].

55. Lifson AR, Thai D, Hang K. Lack of immunization documentation in Minnesota ref-ugees: challenges for refugee preventive health care. J Immigr Health 2001;3(1): 47–52.

56. Evaluating and Updating Immunizations during the Domestic Medical Examina-tion for Newly Arrived Refugees. Centers for Disease Control and Prevention. Available at: https://www.cdc.gov/immigrantrefugeehealth/guidelines/domestic/immunizations-guidelines.html. Accessed April 17, 2020.

57. Willink A, Reed NS, Swenor B, et al. Dental, vision, and hearing services: access, spending, and coverage for medicare beneficiaries: the role medicare advantage plans play in providing dental, vision, and hearing services to older adults, partic-ularly among low-and middle-income beneficiaries. Health Aff 2020;39(2): 297–304.

58. Mertz E, O'Neil E. The growing challenge of providing oral health care services to all Americans. Health Aff 2002;21(5):65–77.

59. Shelley D, Russell S, Parikh NS, et al. Ethnic disparities in self-reported oral health status and access to care among older adults in NYC. J Urban Health 2011;88(4): 651–62.

60. Howard JR, Ramirez J, Li Y, et al. Dental care access for low-income and immi-grant cancer patients in New York City. J Community Health 2015;40(1):110–5.

61. Doucette HJ, Haslam KS, Zelmer KC, et al. The use of language interpreters for immigrant clients in a dental hygiene clinic. Can J Dental Hyg 2018;52(3):167–73. Available at: https://files.cdha.ca/profession/journal/v52n3.pdf#page=9.

62. Brooks K, Stifani B, Batlle HR, et al. Patient perspectives on the need for and bar-riers to professional medical interpretation. R Med J 2016;99(1):30–3.

63. Capozzi BM, Giblin-Scanlon LJ, Rainchuso L. Treatment of a culturally diverse refugee population: dental hygiene students' perceptions and experiences. J Dent Hyg 2018;92(2):50–6.

64. Wilson FA, Wang Y, Stimpson JP, et al. Disparities in visual impairment by immi-grant status in the United States. Am J Ophthalmol 2014;158(4):800–7.e5.

65. Martin SA, Frutiger EA. Vision stations: addressing corrective vision needs with low-cost technologies. Glob Adv Health Med 2015;4(2):46–51.

66. Pape L, Kennedy K, Kaf W, et al. Immigration within the United States: prevalence of childhood hearing loss revisited. Am J Audiol 2014;23(2):238–41.

67. Hughes JD. Hearing loss: etiology, management and societal implications. Hauppauge, NY: Nova Science Publishers; 2016.

68. Masterson EA, Themann CL, Calvert GM. Prevalence of hearing loss among noise-exposed workers within the agriculture, forestry, fishing, and hunting sector, 2003-2012. Am J Ind Med 2018;61(1):42–50.
69. Afanuh S, Kardous CA, National Institute for Occupational Safety and Health. Reducing noise hazards for call and dispatch center operators 2011.
70. Themann C, Suter AH, Stephenson MR. National research agenda for the prevention of occupational hearing loss—Part 2. In: Stephenson MR, editor. Seminars in hearing, vol. 34. New York: Thieme Medical Publishers; 2013. p. 208–52.
71. Rabinowitz PM, Duran R. Is acculturation related to use of hearing protection? AI-HAJ 2001;62(5):611–4.
72. Ramos AK, Fuentes A, Trinidad N. Perception of Job-related risk, training, and use of personal protective equipment (PPE) among Latino immigrant hog CAFO workers in Missouri: a pilot study. Safety (Basel) 2016;2(4):25.
73. Swinkels H, Pottie K, Tugwell P, et al, Canadian Collaboration for Immigrant and Refugee Health (CCIRH). Development of guidelines for recently arrived immigrants and refugees to Canada: Delphi consensus on selecting preventable and treatable conditions. CMAJ 2011;183(12):E928–32.
74. Recommended Adult Immunization Schedule for ages 19 years or older, United States, 2020. Centers for Disease Control and Prevention. 2020. Available at: https://www.cdc.gov/vaccines/schedules/hcp/imz/adult.html. [Accessed 17 April 2020].
75. Chapter 9 - Vaccination Requirement. U.S. Citizenship and Immigration Services. 2019. Available at: https://www.uscis.gov/policy-manual/volume-8-part-b-chapter-9. Accessed August 1, 2020.

Preventive Care in Children and Adolescents

Shruti Simha, MD, MPH[a,b],*, Amy C. Brown, MD, MHS[c]

KEYWORDS

- Immigrant children • Refugee children • Preventive care • Cultural sensitivity

KEY POINTS

- Immigrant children, including refugees, adoptees, undocumented children, unaccompanied minors, and children immigrating with other types of visas, have unique health care needs.
- Immigrant children need timely screening and medical care by providers who are experienced in immigrant health and can provide care with cultural humility.
- Preventive care for immigrant children entails establishing a medical home and providing ongoing care and anticipatory guidance tailored to immigrant families.

BACKGROUND

Overall Scope

The current geopolitical climate has led to record levels of forced migration and displacement of people. According to the United Nations High Commissioner for Refugees (UNHCR), 70.8 million people worldwide have been forced from their homes. Among them are nearly 25.9 million refugees, more than half of whom are less than 18 years old.[1] In the United States, 1 in 4 children (approximately 18.4 million children) lives in an immigrant family. Eighty-nine percent of these children are born in the United States and are US citizens.[2]

Children immigrate to the United States with or without parents for many reasons, including economic or educational pursuits, international adoption, seeking refuge from threatening conditions in their home countries, or even human trafficking.[2] Children may arrive on a temporary visa, have permanent permission to remain in the United States (green card holders or lawful permanent residents), come with refugee status, seek asylum on arrival, or remain without legal status.[2]

[a] Tim and Carolynn Rice Center for Child and Adolescent Health, Cone Health, 301 East Wendover Avenue, Suite 400, Greensboro, NC 27401, USA; [b] Department of Pediatrics, University of North Carolina at Chapel Hill, Chapel Hill, NC, USA; [c] Department of Pediatrics, University of Virginia, PO Box 800386, Charlottesville, VA 22908-0386, USA
* Corresponding author. Tim and Carolynn Rice Center for Child and Adolescent Health, Cone Health, 301 East Wendover Avenue, Suite 400, Greensboro, NC 27401.
E-mail address: shruti.simha@conehealth.com

Prim Care Clin Office Pract 48 (2021) 99–116
https://doi.org/10.1016/j.pop.2020.09.007
0095-4543/21/© 2020 Elsevier Inc. All rights reserved.

Access to Health Care for Immigrant Children

Immigration status is a social determinant of health and can greatly affect access to health care and other resources. Refugees and asylees qualify for Medicaid or Children's Health Insurance Program (CHIP) on arrival to the United States without a wait period. Other lawfully present immigrants may have a 5-year wait period depending on the state.[3] However, undocumented children are not eligible for Medicaid/CHIP or Marketplace health coverage in the United States, with some exceptions for state-funded programs.

Recommendations for Initial Screening of Immigrant Children

The Centers for Disease Control and Prevention (CDC) and American Academy of Pediatrics (AAP) have put forth excellent guidelines for initial screening of immigrant children.[3,4] The AAP also recommends connecting children to a medical home in a timely manner.[5] Although the AAP toolkit is designed for newly arrived refugees and international adoptees, it can be a helpful guide for clinicians caring for other newly arrived immigrant children, including children without legal status in the United States. It is important to remember that children without a legal status often have little to no health surveillance before entering the United States.

Initial Visit Interview and Examination

Providers should request all previous medical records for review and ensure adequate time for the initial visit. The interview involves details of migration, trauma, and possibly family separation, so must be conducted in a sensitive manner, in the presence of trained interpreters. The interview and examination should incorporate trauma-informed approaches and, if necessary, the sensitive parts can be deferred to another visit. It is critical to establish a trusting relationship before exploring trauma. During the physical examination, consider cultural differences and preferences among individual patients and families.

Refer to **Table 1** for guidelines on the initial screening and examination of immigrant children.

Immunizations

Immigrant children are at higher risk for vaccine-preventable diseases because of incomplete vaccine histories, suboptimal serologic responses (caused by vaccine storage issues or malnutrition) or vaccine hesitancy because of misinformation.[13,14]

Unlike US-bound immigrants arriving on certain visas that mandate vaccination before arrival, mandatory vaccination is not required for refugees. However, the overseas vaccination program for US-bound refugees has made it possible for refugees to receive several predeparture, age-appropriate vaccines. Vaccines administered through this program are recorded on DS-3025 (Vaccination Documentation Worksheet) and are compatible with the Advisory Committee on Immunization Practices.[4] Refugees need all the recommended vaccines in order to apply for permanent residency after they have resided in the United States for 1 year. For vaccines recorded in a foreign language, language translations are available in the CDC Pink Book.[15]

Immunization history should be addressed at the initial visit, and children lacking vaccines can be caught up according to CDC guidelines. Often, providers must decide whether to revaccinate or obtain serologic testing. Revaccination is generally preferred for uninsured children without immunization records because of the financial costs of serologic testing. Moreover, excessive immunization rarely causes systemic

Table 1
Guidelines for initial screening and examination of immigrant children

History	• History of migration, including country of origin, country of transit, refugee camp or Office of Refugee Resettlement facility • Birth history, past medical history, surgical history, history of transfusions, tattoos and cultural practices including FGM • Prior medical records and immunizations • Nutrition history and exposure to toxins • Menarche/pubertal history • Sexual history • Substance abuse in patient and family members • Educational history: last grade of school attended, history of learning difficulties; primary language of learning and languages spoken and written at home • Family history: history of HIV, hepatitis B, hepatitis C, tuberculosis • Social history, including family members, immigration status, parental education and employment, community support, food insecurity, housing situation • History of trauma or abuse
Developmental screens	ASQ,[6] PEDS,[7] SWYC,[8] MCHAT-R[9]
Initial mental health screens	PSC,[10] PHQ-9[11] or RHS-15 (>14 y)[12]
Complete physical examination	• Growth parameters, including weight, length, head circumference (in children <2 y), temperature, respiratory rate, heart rate, and blood pressure (children ≥3 y unless warranted for younger ages) • Growth/nutrition: check for physical signs of malnutrition and vitamin deficiencies • Vision/hearing screen • Detailed oral examination • Complete lymph node examination • Thyroid examination for goiter • Skin examination for dermatitis, scars from injuries, abuse, burns/rashes/complimentary medicine scars (burn from sticks, cupping, and coining) • Cardiac examination: consider undiagnosed congenital heart disease and rheumatic valvular disorders • Respiratory examination for pulmonary disease • Abdominal examination to check for splenomegaly or hepatomegaly • Genital examination for FGM

Abbreviations: ASQ, Ages & Stages Questionnaire; FGM, female genital mutilation; HIV, human immunodeficiency virus; MCHAT-R, Modified Checklist for Autism in Toddlers, Revised; PEDS, Parents' Evaluation of Developmental Status; PHQ-9, Patient Health Questionnaire 9; RHS-15, Refugee Health Screener 15; SWYC, Survey of Well-being of Young Children.

Data from American Academy of Pediatrics (AAP). Immigrant Child Health Toolkit. Available at: https://www.aap.org/en-us/advocacy-and-policy/aap-health-initiatives/Immigrant-Child-Health-Toolkit/Pages/Immigrant-Child-Health-Toolkit.aspx. Accessed Feb 22 2020; and Centers for Disease Control and Prevention (CDC). Immigrant and Refugee Health: Guidelines for U.S. domestic medical examination for newly arrived refugees. Available at: https://www.cdc.gov/immigrantrefugeehealth/guidelines/domestic/domestic-guidelines.html. Accessed Feb 22 2020.

adverse effects. The federally funded Vaccines for Children (VFC) program provides free vaccines to all uninsured or underinsured immigrant children.

Refer to **Table 2** for special considerations regarding immunizations.[4]

Recommended Laboratory Tests

The AAP recommends a tiered approach to laboratory screening for foreign-born immigrant children from low-resource countries. Providers should balance the need for testing and subsequent treatment with costs for patients without access to health insurance. The laboratory tests also must be tailored to the country or region of origin and migration history.

Refer to **Box 1** for tiered laboratory screening.[3,4]

Table 2 Special considerations regarding immunizations	
Infections/ Vaccines	**Special Considerations**
• HBV	• HBsAg-positive US-bound refugees are not vaccinated with HBV vaccine • Defer serologic testing for >4 wk after the third and final dose of HBV vaccine to avoid false-positive HBsAg and anti-HBs
• Varicella	• Serologic testing for varicella may be more cost-effective in newly arrived adults compared with children because children may not be infected because of variation in median age of varicella infection worldwide • Administering varicella vaccine to children may be a better option because of availability of the vaccine through VFC
• HAV	• Many immigrant children have been exposed to HAV and are immune • Consider the cost-effectiveness of serologic testing vs immunizing with HAV vaccine
• OPV	• All OPV-using countries switched in April 2016 from trivalent OPV to bivalent OPV, which contains only types 1 and 3 polioviruses. The United States has been using IPV, which contains all 3 polio virus types, since 2000 • CDC recommends children with historical documentation of OPV given in or after April 2016 be revaccinated with IPV[16]
• PCV	• PCV10 and PCV13 are the 2 polysaccharide-protein conjugate vaccines available worldwide since 2019 • PCV13 is the vaccine routinely used in the United States. PPSV23 is only indicated in certain high-risk populations • Previously unvaccinated or incompletely vaccinated immigrant children need to receive catch-up doses of PCV13 per the CDC catch-up immunization schedule. PCV13 can be administered to complete the series in children who have previously received some doses of PCV10[17,18]

Abbreviations: HBsAg, hepatitis B surface antigen; anti-HBs, hepatitis B surface antibody; HAV, hepatitis A virus; HBV, hepatitis B virus; IPV, inactivated polio vaccine; OPV, oral polio vaccine; PCV, pneumococcal conjugate vaccine; PPSV23, pneumococcal polysaccharide vaccine 23.

Data from Centers for Disease Control and Prevention (CDC). Immigrant and Refugee Health: Evaluating and Updating Immunizations during the Domestic Medical Examination for Newly Arrived Refugees. Available at: https://www.cdc.gov/immigrantrefugeehealth/guidelines/domestic/immunizations-guidelines.html. Accessed Feb22 2020.

> **Box 1**
> **Laboratory screening**
>
> *Tiered laboratory testing*
>
> Tier 1
> - Complete blood count with differential to screen for anemia and eosinophilia
> - Lead: children 6 months to 16 years old
> - Tuberculosis testing: tuberculosis skin test for children less than 2 years old, interferon gamma release assays for those 2 years of age and older
> - Hepatitis B surface antigen, hepatitis B core antibody, and hepatitis B surface antibody[4]
> - Intestinal parasite evaluation (if no predeparture treatment records available)[4]
>   - Stool O and P- 3 samples at least 24 hours apart or presumptive treatment with albendazole
>   - *Strongyloides* immunoglobulin (Ig) G or presumptive treatment with ivermectin if more than 15 kg, unless from *Loa loa* endemic country
>   - Schistosoma IgG or presumptive treatment with praziquantel if more than 4 years old and no history of neurocysticercosis
> - Screening for human immunodeficiency virus and syphilis (rapid plasma reagin or Venereal Disease Research Laboratory)[4]
> - Hemoglobin electrophoresis to universally screen for sickle cell trait/disease and thalassemia
>
> Tier 2
> - Newborn screen for infants less than 6 months old
> - Glucose-6-phosphate dehydrogenase activity
> - Thyroid-stimulating hormone in 6 months to 3 years[3]
> - Vitamin deficiency screening
> - Hepatitis C antibody in high-risk cases
> - Urine beta human chorionic gonadotropin
> - Polymerase chain reaction or malaria thin and thick blood smears (×3)or malaria rapid diagnostic test[4]
> - Urine *Neisseria gonorrhoeae/Chlamydia*
>
> *Data from* American Academy of Pediatrics (AAP). Immigrant Child Health Toolkit. Available at: https://www.aap.org/en-us/advocacy-and-policy/aap-health-initiatives/Immigrant-Child-Health-Toolkit/Pages/Immigrant-Child-Health-Toolkit.aspx. Accessed Feb 22 2020; and Centers for Disease Control and Prevention (CDC). Immigrant and Refugee Health: Guidelines for U.S. domestic medical examination for newly arrived refugees. Available at: https://www.cdc.gov/immigrantrefugeehealth/guidelines/domestic/domestic-guidelines.html. Accessed Feb 22 2020.

SPECIAL CONSIDERATIONS FOR THE INITIAL VISIT
Infectious Disease

Infectious diseases are the most common health issues facing newly arrived immigrant children. Chronic malnutrition, limited access to routine health care, endemicity of certain infections, and environmental exposures such as a lack of clean water and/or sanitation put immigrant children at risk. Providers must recognize the clinical manifestations of infections common to immigrant children, routinely screen children at their initial visits, and work in coordination with local health officials and infectious disease specialists to manage all positive children.

For more information on specific childhood infections and treatment recommendations, refer to the AAP Red Book, AAP Immigrant toolkit, and CDC Refugee Health Guidelines.[3,4,19]

Mycobacterium tuberculosis

Tuberculosis (TB) is endemic worldwide, and the incidence of multidrug-resistant TB is increasing.[4] Immigrants account for 50% of new TB cases in the United States.[20]

Strict predeparture guidelines require TB testing for all refugees and international adoptees[4]; however, testing for other immigrant populations is inconsistent. Consequently, all immigrant children should be tested 8 to 12 weeks after arrival. The AAP Redbook recommends tuberculin skin tests (TSTs) for children less than 2 years old and interferon gamma release assays (IGRAs) for children greater than or equal to 2 years old (preferred to TST to avoid false-positive TST results in children who have previously received the bacille Calmette-Guérin [BCG] vaccine).[19] Previous BCG vaccination may affect TST results, but, importantly, it should not influence the interpretation of TST results. Consider retesting immunocompromised and/or malnourished children once their overall health status improves because these factors can lead to false-negative TST/IGRA results.[19] Children with positive TST or IGRA results should undergo a thorough examination and chest radiography to determine active versus latent disease.

Parasitic infections

Some of the most common infections immigrant children encounter are parasitic infections from contaminated soil, water, and food. Many children are asymptomatic at the time of presentation. Other children present with symptoms such as abdominal pain/distension, nausea, vomiting, diarrhea, malabsorption, chronic anemia, failure to thrive, anorexia, papular dermatitis, and/or hematuria.[19] Symptoms depend on the specific infectious cause, and further details can be found in the Kelly Reese and Brianna Moyer's article, "Refugee Medical Screening," in this issue. Providers should obtain stool ova and parasite examinations for symptomatic children and/or children who were not empirically treated before arrival. AAP and CDC recommend obtaining 2 to 3 stool and ova parasite examinations ($\geq$24 hours apart) to increase the sensitivity of accurately identifying a pathogen.[4,19] In certain populations, it may be more cost-effective to empirically treat children greater than 1 year old (without neurologic symptoms concerning for neurocysticercosis) with a single dose of albendazole for soil-transmitted helminths.[4,19] Serology testing is preferred for strongyloidiasis and schistosomiasis.[19] Consider retesting any child with continued poor growth, ongoing or recurrent gastrointestinal symptoms, unexplained anemia, or unexplained eosinophilia even months to years after arrival.

Human immunodeficiency virus and syphilis

Routine prenatal screening for human immunodeficiency virus (HIV) and syphilis varies internationally. Consequently, all immigrant children without documentation of prenatal laboratory tests and/or maternal laboratory tests should undergo HIV and syphilis serologic testing on arrival.[19] Among adolescents, predeparture syphilis testing and treatment are required for those greater than or equal to 15 years old who undergo mandatory medical screening abroad, but HIV testing is no longer required and should be considered in high-risk groups.[4,19] Providers may omit HIV and syphilis testing if prenatal laboratory tests and/or recent maternal results are available, the results are negative, and there is no risk of horizontal transmission.

Hepatitis

Hepatitis B is endemic worldwide, and immigrant children are at increased risk for vertical and horizontal transmission.[19] Acute and chronic hepatitis B infections are still common in parts of Asia, Africa, eastern Europe, and states of the former Soviet Union (ie, Russia and the Ukraine).[19] Predeparture hepatitis B testing is mandatory for refugees but is not required for other immigrant populations. Because routine hepatitis B vaccination and prenatal testing varies worldwide, providers should obtain serologic hepatitis B surface antigen (HBsAg) screening for all immigrant children without documentation of prior testing.[4,19]

Hepatitis C testing should be considered in all adoptees and children with a history of organ transplant, blood transfusion, or positive maternal history.[4]

Growth and Nutrition

Malnutrition is common among immigrant children and refugees. Providers should inquire about dietary habits (including breastfeeding), foods that were available overseas and in transit, any religious/cultural food restrictions, known micronutrient deficiencies, and/or past participation in supplemental feeding programs.[3,4] The CDC and AAP recommend using the World Health Organization (WHO) standardized growth charts for all children less than 2 years old and CDC/National Center for Health Statistics (NCHS) reference growth charts for children more than 2 years old.[3,4] Anthropometric measurements can aid providers in identifying children who are wasted (weight for age), underweight (weight for height), or those with chronic malnutrition and stunting (height for age).[4] Although many immigrant children are undernourished, the prevalence of childhood obesity is increasing worldwide and should be addressed.[4]

Providers should offer ongoing nutritional counseling and track growth longitudinally. Although adequate catch-up growth is typically seen within 6 to 24 months after arrival, providers should consider underlying causes of failure to thrive for undernourished children without improved weight gain within the first 3 months.[4,21]

Globally, iron deficiency is present in half of children living in developing countries and has been associated with developmental delays in young children, cognitive impairment in adolescents, and increased lead absorption and toxicity.[4,22] Other common nutritional deficiencies include vitamin D, thiamine, zinc, niacin, vitamin A, vitamin B_{12}, and iodine.[4]

Environmental Toxins

All children 16 years old or younger and those more than 16 years old with a high concern for lead exposure should be screened on arrival. A single capillary or venous blood level greater than or equal to 5 μg/dL is considered increased and should be reported to local health officials. Capillary blood samples should be confirmed by a venous sample[3,4] (further evaluation of increased levels is discussed in Brittany DiVito and colleagues' article, "Common Hematologic, Nutritional, Asthma/Allergic Conditions and Lead Screening/Management," in this issue).

Complementary Medicine and Cultural Practices

Cultural practices, traditional diets and medications, and the concept of disease and healing vary between countries of origin and even between different ethnic groups from the same region. A few considerations relevant to pediatrics are mentioned here.

Female genital cutting/mutilation

Female genital mutilation (FGM) includes all procedures that involve partial or total removal of the external female genitalia, or other injury to the female genital organs for nonmedical reasons. It is mostly performed on young girls between infancy and adolescence and is mainly concentrated in the western, eastern, and north-eastern regions of Africa, in some countries in the Middle East and Asia, as well as in immigrants from that region.[23] FGM is a violation of human rights and causes significant medical complications. A detailed examination of the genitalia is therefore vital during the initial visit.

Coining and cupping

Coining (cao gio) is a common practice in Southeast Asia for treatment of minor illnesses such as flu, cold, headaches, fever, and low energy. During this process, the skin is lubricated with heated oil and then scraped with a ceramic spoon, coin, or metal cap. Cupping is another ancient practice involving circular suction cups made of glass, bamboo, or earthenware that are applied to the skin to treat pain. These practices, also used in infants and children, can cause superficial burns, bruises, and hematomas and could be misinterpreted as abuse.[24]

Herbs and spices

Herbs and other compounds used worldwide may be contaminated with lead and other metals. For example, turmeric, often used in cooking and for medicinal purposes, and traditional eye cosmetics (containing kohl, kajal, or surma), have both been associated with childhood lead exposure and poisoning.[25,26] For children who have increased lead levels, a detailed history of herbal and eye cosmetic use (for boys and girls) should be obtained.

Oral Health

Oral health is a significant health issue for most newly arrived immigrants. Cultural beliefs, language barriers, misunderstandings regarding preventive oral health, and a lack of dental coverage are common barriers to care. Certain immigrant groups are disproportionately affected, including those who had limited access to care in their home countries or with certain dietary/feeding practices. The NCHS data from 2015 to 2016 showed that Hispanic children had the highest prevalence of dental caries in the United States.[27] In contrast, East African children had lower rates of dental caries, likely related to traditional diets low in sugar and cultural practices such as the use of chewing sticks.[28]

Early childhood caries is associated with significant morbidity (chronic pain, poor feeding, infection, teeth crowding, self-esteem issues) and economic costs (missed school, increased emergency room visits, costly dental procedures).[29] Many immigrant families do not access dental care for children unless they are in pain and may not recognize the importance of caring for primary teeth. Although children who are eligible for Medicaid have dental coverage until 21 years of age, few dental offices accept Medicaid, making access to care difficult. Immigrant families need counseling regarding preventive dental care, prompt referral to a dental home, and, when appropriate, fluoride application.

Development

Early childhood development is affected by a multitude of factors, including genetics, biology, family, and environment. Migration has a significant impact on the development of children and differences in cultural practices, parenting practices, and language barriers make it exceedingly difficult to evaluate and detect developmental and behavioral problems in young immigrant children.

The AAP recommends using age-appropriate developmental screens for initial and subsequent visits.[3] Commonly used screens include the Ages & Stages Questionnaire (ASQ), Parents' Evaluation of Developmental Status (PEDS), and the Survey of Well-being of Young Children (SWYC).[6–8]

The ASQ is an in-depth, 1-step screen for children 1 to 66 months old. It is available in 6 languages and takes 10 to 15 minutes to complete. It has the highest sensitivity (86%) and specificity (85%) among developmental screens used in children.[6]

The PEDS tool can be used for children less than or equal to 8 years old. It is ideal for families with limited English proficiency because it is available in more than 50 languages and is designed to be fast, accurate, and simple (completed in 3–6 minutes).[7]

The SWYC screening tool is for children 2 to 60 months old and is available on the Floating Hospital for Children Web site.[8] It is available in 10 languages and addresses social determinants of health in addition to development and behavior. It takes less than 15 minutes to complete and has a sensitivity (76%) and specificity (77%) comparable with PEDS but lower than ASQ.[7]

School Readiness

Like difficulties in screening for developmental delays, screening for learning disabilities among immigrant children can be challenging. Culturally competent testing in other languages is lacking and most standardized assessment tools do not account for bilingualism.[30] As a result, English language learners (ELLs) are frequently placed in inappropriate learning environments.[31]

Time and resource constraints for school personnel may further this problem. Personnel often receive inadequate training in cross-cultural education, second language acquisition, and ELL education, adding to the difficulty in addressing learning issues among immigrant children.

Mental Health

Although children are extremely resilient, immigrating to the United States can be a challenging experience. Children not only experience trauma in their countries of origin (exposure to violence, oppression, poverty) but during transit (separation from caregivers, disruption in education, witnessed traumatic events, abuse) and on resettlement (prolonged detention, acculturation stress, discrimination, fear).[2,32] Acculturation stress can occur as children adapt to a new language, educational system, and cultural expectations while also navigating a new identity, intergenerational conflicts, or parental reunification after prolonged separation.[2,33] Undocumented immigrants and children living in mixed legal status homes may live under the constant threat of deportation.[2] These threats have been associated with poor school performance, increased school dropout rates, and decreased access to health care.[3] Immigrant children may experience cultural prejudice, racial discrimination, or bullying. Adverse experiences are cumulative and can have a negative impact on the intellectual, social, emotional, and physical development of children.[34] Consequently, many immigrant children have anxiety; depression; posttraumatic stress disorder (PTSD); and occasionally somatization, sleep disturbance, and substance abuse.[2,4,33]

Providers, with the help of medically trained interpreters, should screen for signs/symptoms of emotional and behavioral conditions and provide immediate and ongoing referrals to integrated mental health providers, community-based support organizations, and/or school-based interventions.[3] A strengths-based, trauma-informed approach and understanding risk and protective factors that affect immigrant children on individual, familial, community, and societal levels are vital.[33] Studies have shown that attachment to at least 1 caring adult can greatly buffer the effects of adverse childhood experiences.[34] Thus providers must foster caregiver resilience and support as they care for their children.

Refer to **Table 1** for a list of psychosocial screening tools that have been validated in cross-cultural situations.

Special Populations

Unaccompanied minors

Since 2014, US Customs and Border Protection (CBP) agents have seen a dramatic increase in the number of unaccompanied immigrant children attempting to cross the southern US border. Migrant children are considered unaccompanied if they are less than 18 years old and are not accompanied by an adult who is verifiably the biological parent or child's legal guardian at the time of detention. Most of these migrants are from El Salvador, Guatemala, Honduras, and Mexico.[35] More than 76,000 unaccompanied children were detained while attempting to enter the United States from October 2018 to September 2019 alone.[35] Many of these children are seeking asylum from violence, poverty, abuse, and/or economic instability in their home countries.[32,36] Other children desire to be reunified with family members residing in the United States.

Unaccompanied children are initially held in CBP processing centers but, by law, must be transferred to shelters supervised by the Office of Refugee Resettlement (ORR) within 72 hours of arrival.[32,37] Individual ORR shelters are responsible for overseeing their medical care while in detention, although the care and services offered to children vary by facility.[32,37] The average stay is 66 days.[38] Unaccompanied children are then released to community sponsors (parents, adult family members, or nonfamily individuals who have been vetted and approved by the government) throughout the United States while awaiting deportation hearings.[37]

US providers need to be aware of the unique risks and medical needs of unaccompanied children. Similar to other immigrant children, unaccompanied children may experience significant disruptions in their education, exposure to trauma, and separation from family members. However, in contrast with accompanied minors, they are at a particular risk for sexual assault, exploitation, and victimization because of a lack of parental protection.[36] During the process of resettlement, they may struggle with reunification, isolation, and acculturation. These stressors lead to higher levels of anxiety, depression, and PTSD among unaccompanied minors because they lack the buffering relationships that are important for maintaining psychological resilience and reducing toxic stress.[2,34]

Children without representation are 5 times more likely to be denied asylum in the United States.[39] Providers should connect unaccompanied children to medical-legal partnerships and pro bono legal advocates who can aid them through the immigration process.[2] Many children are eligible for asylum through special immigrant juvenile visas or additional nonimmigrant visas if they have been victims of human trafficking (T visas) or other serious crimes (U visas).[2]

Children at risk for human trafficking

Human trafficking (HT) is an increasingly acknowledged global health crisis affecting individuals in every country and in every region of the world. At any given time, 2.5 million individuals are at risk for trafficking worldwide, and between 244,000 and 325,000 children remain at risk each year in the United States alone.[40] More than one-third of all HT victims are children.[41]

HT is defined as the "recruiting, harboring, transporting, providing, or obtaining a person for compelled labor or commercial sex acts through the use of force, fraud or coercion."[42] The most predominant form of HT is sexual exploitation, although other forms of exploitation (forced labor, domestic servitude, forced child labor, and the use of child soldiers) are increasingly recognized.[43] Commercial sexual exploitation of children involves engaging minors (<18 years of age) in sexual acts for items of value (food, shelter, drugs, money, or other basic necessities) and may or may not involve force, fraud, or coercion.[44]

Immigrant children are at particular risk for HT. Victims rarely self-identify because of shame or guilt, fear of retribution from their traffickers, fear of arrest, drug addiction, lack of knowledge that they are victims, or, in cases of undocumented immigration, fear of deportation.[40,44] They may experience injuries from violence, sexually transmitted infections, and other reproductive health issues, poorly controlled chronic health conditions, substance abuse, depression, anxiety, and PTSD.[40,44]

Table 3 lists some history and examination findings that are considered risk factors for HT.

Providers should be familiar with mandatory reporting laws, federal and state laws protecting HT victims, and national antitrafficking advocacy organizations such as the Polaris Project (www.polarisproject.org/), Shared Hope International (www.sharedhope.org/) and HEAL (Health, Education, Advocacy, Linkage) Trafficking (www.healtrafficking.org/). The National Human Trafficking Resource Hotline (1-888-373-7888) is available 24/7 to assist providers with local resources.[45] Specialized nonimmigrant (T) visas may provide immigration relief to transnational victims of severe forms of sex and labor trafficking.[2]

ONGOING MEDICAL FOLLOW-UP
Anticipatory Guidance

Most immigrant children have previously only seen a health care provider for sick visits or emergencies and need to understand the importance of preventive care. Providers should also consider barriers such as language difficulty and lack of transportation when addressing compliance with medical appointments.

Anticipatory guidance is a critical part of pediatric well visits. This guidance needs to be delivered in culturally sensitive ways, understanding that other cultures often value

---

Table 3
History and examination findings that are considered risk factors for human trafficking

Historical Factors	Physical Examination Findings
• Childhood maltreatment (abuse/neglect)	• Fearful and withdrawn child
• Involvement with Child Protective Services, foster care, juvenile detention, or gangs	• Accompanied by an unrelated, domineering adult
• Runaway and homeless youth	• Physical injuries from violence
• Substance misuse	• Tattoos (sexually explicit, gang affiliations)
• Behavioral/mental health problems	• Sexually transmitted infections
• Developmental/learning difficulties	• Signs of substance misuse
• LGBTQ youth	• Poor dentition or poorly controlled chronic conditions
• Recurrent sexually transmitted infections, unwanted pregnancy or abortion	
• Parental mental health disorder, intimate partner violence, or substance misuse	
• Living in an area with poverty, a transient male population, or local prostitution	

Adapted from Brown AC, Barron CE. Human trafficking. Pediatr Rev 2018;39(2):102-103; and Greenbaum J, Crawford-Jakubiak JE. Child sex trafficking and commercial sexual exploitation: Health care needs of victims. Pediatrics 2015;135(3):566-574; with permission.

interdependence and collective decision making more than personal autonomy and independence.

Refer to **Table 4** for age-appropriate anticipatory guidance for well visits.

Guidance specific to adolescents follows.

Bullying

Although bullying is prevalent among all children, immigrant and refugee children are more likely to experience bullying related to religious, cultural, or racial factors. Even among the same ethnic group, immigrant children are more likely to be bullied than native-born children. Racism, anti-immigrant sentiments, and religious and political rhetoric affect bullying.[49]

Providers should address this important topic with immigrant parents and offer guidance on recognizing signs of bullying in their children and tools to deal with and report bullying at school. It is important to discuss with parents the risks of cyber bullying and the need for setting boundaries with technology.[50]

Sexual health

In many cultures and religions, sexual health is a taboo subject and even friendships with teens of the opposite sex may be discouraged. However, it is important for providers to ask parents and adolescents about their values and beliefs regarding dating and relationships.

During the visit, providers should interview teenagers alone and explain adolescent confidentiality. These conversations can take place at future visits after establishing a trusting relationship. Providers should discuss with teens issues such as safe sex, contraception, sexual consent, intimate partner violence, and the dangers of HT. Parents and adolescents may benefit from discussions on cultural norms in the West (clothing, drugs, dating, sexual relationships) and how to protect against undue influences.

Treatment and Referrals

Treatment

Treatment largely depends on the examination and laboratory findings, but all newly arrived immigrant children should receive a standard treatment plan as follows:

- Catch-up vaccines per CDC schedule with a follow-up plan. If TSTs are placed, they can either be placed with live vaccines or greater than or equal to 4 weeks after live vaccines.
- Multivitamin with iron for all children 6 months to 5 years old and children more than 5 years old with poor nutrition.
- Fluoride varnish for children less than 5 years old.
- Adolescent counseling and contraception as appropriate.
- Establish medical home and primary care provider, and set follow-up appointments.

Referrals

- Women, infants, and children referral (infants and children <5 years old, pregnant women)
- Care coordination with local agencies and school
- Dental referral: for uninsured children, local health departments (or clinics with a sliding fee) may be an option
- Referral for developmental evaluation and therapies as needed
- Mental health referrals as needed
- Subspecialty referrals for underlying medical conditions

Table 4
Age-appropriate anticipatory guidance

	Nutrition	Oral Health	Safety	Sleep	Development
Infancy	Stress importance of breastfeeding Breastfeeding is common until age 2–4 y in some cultures[46] Discuss timing of solid food introduction and concept of baby foods in the United States Encourage home-cooked foods No water until 6 mo of age and no juice until 12 mo of age Address home remedies for colic	Discuss bottle caries and avoidance of prolonged bottle use or nighttime feeds in older infants	Discuss sudden infant death syndrome, back to sleep, and the safe use of bassinets and cribs Discuss the need for infant supervision by older teens and adults rather than younger siblings	Cosleeping is common in most cultures other than Western culture. Letting the baby or young child sleep alone may be viewed as a sign of child neglect Room sharing rather than bed sharing is a helpful way of negotiating this issue[47]	Read and talk to baby in native languages and English if able
Early childhood	Encourage family meals and home cooking Discuss harms of processed and junk foods	Introduce the concept of preventive dental visits and brushing teeth twice daily with fluoride toothpaste	Educate about poison control Car safety and use of car seats[4] Discuss need for child supervision and laws regarding age for babysitting Positive parenting, discipline, and avoiding physical punishment Discuss US laws around child abuse and neglect	Discuss importance of sleep hygiene and bedtime routine for children but know that many cultures do not practice strict bedtime routines and allow children to fall asleep naturally[48]	Encourage early literacy by reading daily or storytelling in native language if parents are unable to read Avoid television and other screens until age 2 y and limit screen time to 1 h for ages 2–5 y Encourage enrollment in Head Start programs

(continued on next page)

Table 4
(continued)

	Nutrition	Oral Health	Safety	Sleep	Development
Elementary school age and adolescence	Address healthy eating and lifestyle and importance of family meals Encourage milk intake with 2–3 daily servings of dairy	Discuss harmful effects of refined sugar and carbohydrates on dental health. Traditional diets are low in sugar and beneficial for superior dental health	Introduce concept of safety equipment such as helmets for biking and skating Address car seat safety and need for use of forward-facing car seat or booster Children younger than 13 y need to sit in the back seat Discuss Internet safety and parental monitoring and safety checks	Stress importance of sleep in school-aged children and the need to maintain consistent bedtime Avoid screen time before bedtime	School: Educate parents about the US school system and need to advocate for their children Inform parents that all children in the United States have access to free education regardless of immigration status Discuss special education and learning disabilities
Adolescence	Encourage teens to be involved in meal planning to ensure healthy nutrition and lifestyle	Discuss importance of flossing in addition to regular brushing	Discuss safety and rules regarding driving in teenagers, and avoidance of drugs, alcohol, smoking, and vaping Discuss risks involving unsupervised Internet use	Remind teens that their need for sleep increases in adolescence even though there is sleep latency in teenagers	Discuss career plans and resources such as school guidance counselors

SUMMARY

This article provides a summary of the guidelines for preventive care in newly arrived immigrant children and adolescents but can also be used for ongoing medical care. It is important to consider the unique challenges faced by this population to help close the health equity gap. The COVID-19 (coronavirus disease 2019) pandemic has now widened the health equity gap and exposed weaknesses in the US health care system.[51] Now more than ever, clinicians need to strengthen community-based interventions and advocate for local, state, and national policy changes to support the health and well-being of immigrant children.

CLINICS CARE POINTS

- Assess for malnutrition in all immigrant children. Current guidelines recommend using the WHO standardized growth charts for children less than 2 years old.[3,4] Children who appear to have short stature or are underweight on the CDC growth curve may be in a healthy range on the WHO growth curve.

- Evaluate for developmental delays using age-appropriate screens. Be alert for learning difficulties in school-aged immigrant children because standardized assessment tools may not account for language and cultural differences.

- Provide universal mental health screening to immigrant children using cross-culturally validated tools with a strengths-based, trauma-informed approach.

- Be aware of the risks of HT among immigrant children and know the mandatory reporting laws and resources available to providers.

DISCLOSURE

The authors have nothing to disclose.

REFERENCES

1. UN Refugee agency (UNHCR) USA. Figures at a glance. Available at: https://www.unhcr.org/figures-at-a-glance.html. Accessed May 9, 2020.
2. Linton JM, Green A, Council on Community Pediatrics. Providing care for children in immigrant families. Pediatrics 2019;144(3):e20192077.
3. AAP immigrant child health toolkit. Available at: https://www.aap.org/en-us/advcy-and-policy/aap-health-initiatives/Immigrant-Child-Health-Toolkit/Pages/Immigrant-Child-Health-Toolkit.aspx. Accessed February 22, 2020.
4. CDC. Guidelines for U.S. domestic medical examination for newly arrived refugees. Available at: https://www.cdc.gov/immigrantrefugeehealth/guidelines/domestic/domestic-guidelines.html. Accessed February 22, 2020.
5. AAP council on community pediatrics. Providing care for immigrant, migrant, and border children. Pediatrics 2013;131(6):e2028–34.
6. Ages and stages questionnaire (ASQ). Brooks publishing company. Available at: http://agesandstages.com. Accessed March 15, 2020.
7. Parents' evaluation of developmental status (PEDS). Frances page glascoe. Available at: http://www.pedstest.com/default.aspx. Accessed March 15, 2020.
8. Survey of wellbeing of young children (SWYC). Floating hospital for children at tufts medical center. Available at: http://www.theswyc.org. Accessed March 15, 2020.

9. Modified checklist for autism in toddlers (M-CHAT). Diana Robins, Deborah Fein, & Marianne Barton. Available at: https://m-chat.org/en-us/page/take-m-chat-test/print-version. Accessed on May 9, 2020.

10. Pediatric symptom checklist (PSC). Massachusetts general hospital. Available at: https://www.massgeneral.org/psychiatry/treatments-and-services/pediatric-symptom-checklist. Accessed May 9, 2020.

11. Patient health questionnaire (PHQ) screeners. Pfizer. Available at: https://www.phqscreeners.com/select-screener. Accessed May 9, 2020.

12. Refugee health screener (RHS-15). Available at: http://refugeehealthta.org/wp-content/uploads/2012/09/RHS15_Packet_PathwaysToWellness-1.pdf. Accessed May 9, 2020.

13. Shetty AK. Infectious diseases among refugee children. Children (Basel) 2019; 6(12):129.

14. Wolff ER, Madlon-Kay DJ. Childhood vaccine beliefs reported by Somali and non-Somali parents. J Am Board Fam Med 2014;27(4):458–64.

15. CDC. Foreign language terms; aids to translating foreign immunization records. Available at: https://www.cdc.gov/vaccines/pubs/pinkbook/downloads/appendices/B/foreign-products-tables.pdf. Accessed May 10, 2020.

16. Marin M, Patel M, Oberste S, et al. Guidance for assessment of poliovirus vaccination status and vaccination of children who have received poliovirus vaccine outside the United States. MMWR Morb Mortal Wkly Rep 2017;66(1):23–5.

17. World health organization (WHO). Available at: https://www.who.int/immunization/policy/position_papers/who_pp_pcv_2019_summary.pdf. Accessed July 9, 2020.

18. CDC. Immunization schedules. Available at: https://www.cdc.gov/vaccines/schedules/hcp/imz/catchup.html#note-pneumo. Accessed July 9, 2020.

19. AAP. Committee on Infectious Diseases. In: Kimberlin DW, Brady MT, Jackson MA, et al, editors. Medical Evaluation for Infectious Diseases for Internationally Adopted, Refugee, and Immigrant Children, pg 194-201, Red Book: 2015 report of the committee on infectious diseases. 31st edition. Elk Grove Village (IL): AAP; 2018.

20. Jenista JA. The immigrant, refugee, or internationally adopted child. Pediatr Rev 2001;22(12):419–29.

21. Hervey K, Vargas D, Klesges L, et al. Overweight among refugee children after arrival in the United States. J Health Care Poor Underserved 2009;20(1):246–56.

22. AAP. Committee on Nutrition. In: Kleinman RE, Greer FR, editors. Chapter 18: Iron pg 405-406. Pediatric nutrition handbook. 7th edition. Elk Grove Village (IL): AAP; 2014.

23. World Health Organization (WHO). Fact sheets: female genital mutilation 2020. Available at: https://www.who.int/news-room/fact-sheets/detail/female-genital-mutilation. Accessed May 22, 2020.

24. Vitale SA, Prashad T. Cultural awareness: coining and cupping. Int Arch Nurs Health Care 2017;3:080.

25. Cowell W, Ireland T, Vorhees D, et al. Ground turmeric as a source of lead exposure in the United States. Public Health Rep 2017;132(3):289–93.

26. Keosaian J, Venkatesh T, D'Amico S, et al. Blood lead levels of children using traditional Indian medicine and cosmetics. Glob Adv Health Med 2019;8. 2164956119870988.

27. Fleming E, Aul J. Prevalence of total and untreated dental caries among youth: US. 2015–2016; NCHS Data Brief, no 307. Hyattsville (MD), USA: National Center for Health Statistics; 2018.

28. Crespo E. The importance of oral health in immigrant and refugee children. Children 2019;6(9):102.
29. AAP. Committee on Nutrition. In: Kleinman RE, Greer FR, editors. Chapter 48: Nutrition and Oral Health, pg 1045-1046. Pediatric nutrition handbook. 7th edition. Elk Grove Village (IL): AAP; 2014.
30. Zehr M. Bilingual students with disabilities get special help. Education Week November 7, 2001. Available at: http://www.ldonline.org/article/13074/. Accessed May 10, 2020.
31. Hamayan EV, Marler B, Sanchez-Lopez C, et al. Reasons for the misidentification of special needs among ELLs 2007. Available at: http://www.ldonline.org/article/40715/. Accessed May 10, 2020.
32. Linton JM, Griffin M, Shapiro AJ. Council on community pediatrics. Detention of immigrant children. Pediatrics 2017;139(5):e20170483.
33. Fazel M, Reed RV, Panter-Brick C, et al. Mental health of displaced and refugee children resettled in high-income countries: risk and protective factors. Lancet 2012;379:266–82.
34. Garner AS, Shonkoff JP. Committee on psychosocial aspects of child and family health; committee on early childhood, adoption, and dependent care; section on developmental and behavioral pediatrics. Early childhood adversity, toxic stress, and the role of the pediatrician: translating developmental science into lifelong health. Pediatrics 2012;129(1):e232–46.
35. US Customs and Border Protection (CBP). Southwest border unaccompanied children apprehensions. Available at: https://www.cbp.gov/newsroom/stats/sw-border-migration/usbp-sw-border-apprehensions-fy2019. Accessed May 11, 2020.
36. UN Refugee Agency (UNHCR). Children on the run, unaccompanied children leaving Central America and Mexico and the need for international protection. Washington, DC: UNHCR 2014. Available at: https://www.unhcr.org/en-us/56fc266f4.pdf. Accessed May 20, 2020.
37. US Department of Health and Human Services. Office of refugee resettlement (ORR). Unaccompanied children's services. Available at: https://www.acf.hhs.gov/orr/resource/unaccompanied-childrens-services. Accessed May 11, 2020.
38. US Department of Health and Human Services. Office of refugee resettlement (ORR). Facts and data. Available at: https://www.acf.hhs.gov/orr/about/ucs/facts-and-data. Accessed May 20, 2020.
39. Kids in Need of Defense (KIND). No child should appear in immigration court alone. Washington, DC: kids in need of defense 2018. Available at: https://supportkind.org/resources/kind-fact-sheet/. Accessed May 20, 2020.
40. American Professional Society on the Abuse of Children (APSAC). The commercial sexual exploitation of children: the medical provider's role in identification, assessment and treatment: APSAC practice guidelines. Chicago, IL: APSAC 2013. Available at: https://docs.wixstatic.com/ugd/4700a8_dff52e3f98e04f02b25d9623619402e8.pdf. Accessed May 5, 2020.
41. UN Office on Drugs and Crime (UNODC). Global report on trafficking in persons 2018. Vienna, Austria: UNODC 2018. Available at: https://www.unodc.org/documents/data-and-analysis/glotip/2018/GLOTiP_2018_BOOK_web_small.pdf. Accessed May 10, 2020.
42. US Department of State (USDOS). Trafficking in persons report. Washington, DC: USDOC 2019. Available at: https://www.state.gov/wp-content/uploads/2019/06/2019-Trafficking-in-Persons-Report.pdf. Accessed May 5, 2020.
43. Brown AC, Barron CE. Human trafficking. Pediatr Rev 2018;39(2):102–3.

44. Greenbaum J, Crawford-Jakubiak JE. Child sex trafficking and commercial sexual exploitation: health care needs of victims. Pediatrics 2015;135(3):566–74.
45. National human trafficking hotline. Available at: https://humantraffickinghotline. org. Accessed May 10, 2020.
46. Bridging refugee youth and children's services (BRYCS). Available at: https:// brycs.org/wp-content/uploads/2018/08/handbook-supporting-early-learning-and-healthy-development-1.pdf. Accessed March 3, 2020.
47. Shimizu M, Park H, Greenfield PM. Infant sleeping arrangements and cultural values among contemporary Japanese mothers. Front Psychol 2014;5:718.
48. Johnson L, Radesky J, Zuckerman B. Cross-cultural parenting: reflections on autonomy and interdependence. Pediatrics 2013;131(4):631–3.
49. Maynard BR, Vaughn MG, Salas-Wright CP, et al. Bullying victimization among school-aged immigrant youth in the United States. J Adolesc Health 2016; 58(3):337–44.
50. American Psychological Association. How parents, teachers and kids can take action to prevent bullying 2011. Available at: http://www.apa.org/helpcenter/ bullying. Accessed March 5, 2020.
51. Page KR, Venkataramani M, Beyrer C, et al. Undocumented U.S. immigrants and covid-19. N Engl J Med 2020;382(21):e62.

Women's Health and Gender-Specific Considerations

Alison N. Huffstetler, MD[a],*, Sarah I. Ramirez, MD[b], Sarah N. Dalrymple, MD[c],
Megan H. Mendez Miller, DO[b]

KEYWORDS

- Immigrant women's health • Refugees • Women's health
- Menstrual practices and beliefs • Contraceptive beliefs • Family planning
- Pregnancy • Female genital mutilation

KEY POINTS

- Menarche is often a significant traditional demarcation for immigrant girls in the transition to becoming a woman. Discuss menstrual practices, how to use common feminine hygiene, and contraception with girls approaching the age of menarche.
- There are significant unmet contraceptive needs among refugees and immigrants as well as several barriers to contraception both before and after arrival in the United States. Ask open-ended questions to determine individual goals for family planning.
- Female genital mutilation (FGM) is a common practice in Africa and the Middle East; inquire about past experiences with FGM because it might affect menstruation, child birth, intercourse, and cervical cancer screening.

INTRODUCTION

Immigrant and refugee women face challenges on arrival in the United States that should be addressed by health care professionals. Clinicians must address women's health topics in a sensitive manner that accommodates differences in background, understanding of health, and beliefs about the medical community. Once a clinician has developed rapport and explored the patient's background, consider discussions regarding contraception, family planning, menstruation, and preventive care. This

Conflicts of interest: None to report.
Financial disclosure: None to report.
[a] Department of Family Medicine and Population Health, Virginia Commonwealth University, 830 East Main Street, Richmond, VA 23219, USA; [b] Department of Family and Community Medicine, Penn State Health, Milton S. Hershey Medical Center, 500 University Drive, Hershey, PA 17033, USA; [c] Department of Family Medicine, University of Virginia, PO Box 800729, Charlottesville, VA 22908, USA
* Corresponding author.
E-mail address: alison.huffstetler@vcuhealth.org

Prim Care Clin Office Pract 48 (2021) 117–129
https://doi.org/10.1016/j.pop.2020.09.008
primarycare.theclinics.com

article addresses experiences that women may have faced around the world that affect their interaction and engagement with the health care system.

CULTURAL CONSIDERATIONS

An Iranian non–English-speaking woman and her 6-year-old daughter arrived at the clinic. After attempting to communicate unsuccessfully with the front desk staff, the family grew distressed. A male staff member placed his hand on the woman's shoulder. She pulled away quickly, stumbling, and fell backward onto the floor. He then extended his hand to aid the fallen woman and she quickly covered her face.

Navigating the Health Care System/Acculturation

Cultural humility is required in order to provide culturally responsive care and acknowledge cultural needs and expectations of the patients. If beliefs of the patients are violated, health care delivery may be negatively affected; specifically, this may result in the patients not expressing their needs or not seeking care at all.[1] For many refugees, there is an expectation that physicians will cure all ailments immediately. Others may delay care as they believe illness is simply a part of life. Incongruent beliefs between patient and clinician prove challenging to health care clinicians, which increases psychological stress of both parties.[2]

Refugees face barriers to accessing care; language is the most commonly cited barrier to care.[3] For many immigrants, English as a second language not only makes it difficult to navigate the health care system but also makes communicating with service clinicians challenging.

Refusal of Male Care

A common barrier is avoidance of male medical clinicians. This avoidance may contribute to health disparities. For many cultures, female modesty is paramount and avoidance of physical contact with men is strictly enforced. These principles may extend to medical care. Refusal of male clinicians may be based on social norms of segregating sexes because of religious beliefs; not facilitating requests for a female clinician may result in profound psychological trauma. Beyond this, for victims of gender-related violence, refugee women may carry an increased burden of mental health disease related to the trauma of past victimization. Clinicians should strive to avoid interactions that may be perceived as threatening to the patient.

Assessment of Religion and Knowledge/Attitudes/Beliefs

Religious persecution is a common reason for fleeing to the host country. Approximately 37% of the refugees admitted to the United States in 2016 were members of religious minorities in their home countries.[4] **Table 1** outlines several religions and examples of the cultural impact that religion may have on women's health. Clinicians should inquire about a woman's religion and incorporate religious beliefs, as appropriate, into the treatment plan.

BEFORE ARRIVAL IN THE UNITED STATES

Each woman has individual experiences with regard to her own health. The conditions in a woman's home country greatly affect her health practices. Cultural perceptions of health, wellness, and disease, as well as the process of immigration or seeking refuge, affect each woman's general and gender-specific health. For example, refugees are more likely than immigrants to have had an unexpected departure from their home countries, and may have spent time in a refugee camp. Especially when fleeing areas

Table 1
World religions and related regions with examples of cultural or religious impact on women's role and/or health

Religion/ Culture	Countries Represented	Example
Islam	Jordan Pakistan Bangladesh Syria Iran Egypt	Women are viewed as a stranger by their families until they birth a male child. After this birth, they are renamed um, meaning mother of, followed by the son's name. If the firstborn is a girl, there is pressure for a quick second pregnancy in hopes for a male infant. After a male birth, the woman is integrated into her family
Christianity	Egypt Ethiopia Kenya Burkina Faso	Female genital mutilation continues to be celebrated in some Christian communities, justified by elders as a traditional practice
Hinduism	China Nepal	Some traditional texts emphasize that women should be honored but not encouraged to think for themselves. Karma theory accepts suffering (such as intimate partner violence) as a payment for sins of prior lives. Violence is permitted or viewed with complacency. Women from Nepal or West Bengal report restrictions in attending religious functions, cooking, and physical contact with others caused because of cultural expectations
Judaism	Israel	Haredi women, the ultraorthodox, have significantly lower rates of mammography and colonoscopy compared with other Jewish and secular women
Buddhism	Thailand-Burma (Myanmar)	Emergency contraception is only available in cases of rape. Traditional beliefs support that life begins with conception, therefore all forms of contraception are stigmatized
Folk religions	Eastern Indonesia	The Nage people believe that health problems and abnormalities in adults are often related to poor food choices of lactating mothers when they were infants

of conflict, refugee women are more vulnerable to sexual assault and exploitation. Through a systematic review of available literature, Gagnon and colleagues[5] broadly categorized the health challenges experienced by refugee women in transit or in camps into:

1. Fertility regulation (ie, changes to fertility patterns)
2. Sexually transmitted infections
3. Sex-based and gender-based violence
4. Pregnancy and childbirth, including loss
5. Health services availability and use

Setting up the Initial Visit

For refugees, health screening on arrival is a required part of the resettlement process (see the Kelly Reese and Brianna Moyer's article, "Refugee Medical Screening," in this issue), but the patient may have specific goals. Assess the patient's goals for establishing and continuing health care as well as her perception of her own health and any conditions she might have. Consider obtaining a thorough gynecologic and obstetric history, including menstrual history and sexual history. Also ask whether she has had any gynecologic examinations previously. Clinicians should be specific with questions and vocabulary to minimize cultural and language barriers. It may be appropriate to delay potentially traumatic questioning until rapport has been built, unless pertinent to an active condition.

WOMEN'S PREVENTIVE CARE

There are several gender-specific considerations when addressing preventive care with female refugees and immigrants (see the articles by Simha and colleagues and Payton and colleagues, in this issue). Many women arriving in the United States have a history of sexual violence and trauma; thus breast and pelvic examinations may not be desired. Female genital mutilation (FGM), discussed later in this article, may also make examinations physically and mentally distressing. On building rapport with these patients, explore their beliefs and values with regard to cancer screening. Offer cervical cancer screening for eligible women and provide risks and benefits for screening. Women more than 65 years of age without prior screening may benefit from 1-time screening. Breast cancer screening should be addressed in a similar fashion, recognizing that rates of breast cancer vary around the world and some women face greater risk (19.3 cases per 100,000 women in eastern Africa vs 89.7 cases per 100,000 women in western Europe).[6] In addition, rates of screening for chronic diseases and cancer vary across countries, which likely contributes to lower incidence of chronic disease and cancer in African countries.[6] Vitamin D screening, which does not currently have enough evidence to be recommended as routine screening for all women, should be considered for those women who wear face and body covering, such as hijabs. In addition, screening for social determinants of health, also not yet recommended by the US Preventive Services Task Force, should be considered using a tool such as the Protocol for Responding to and Addressing Patients Assets, Risks, and Experiences (PREPARE).[7]

MENARCHE AND MENSTRUAL PRACTICES

Menarche signifies the start of the female reproductive years and often marks the transition to full adult status in society. A worldwide trend of earlier age for menarche in both developed and less developed countries has been shown over the last few decades.[8] Many religions and cultures have different views on menarche and what this rite of passage means. For example, many traditional cultural practices in South Asia define menarche as a time when parents withdraw their daughter from school in order to be married.[9]

Several studies show that, although most girls are aware of menstruation before menarche, most girls do not fully understand the physical process of menstruation. A survey of 160 girls in West Bengal found that 68% were aware about menstruation before menarche, but 98% did not know the source of menstrual bleeding. A common belief among Gujjar girls, a seminomadic tribal group in Jammu and Kashmir, is that menstruation is the removal of bad blood from the body necessary to prevent infection.[10]

In less developed countries, there exists a connection between poor menstrual hygiene and higher absenteeism or early dropout rates in adolescent girls, related to lack of privacy, adequate water resources, and proper sanitary disposal at school. However, these cultural norms and experiences continue after migration despite having adequate water, privacy, and disposal resources. Because use of unsanitary reusable menstrual products (eg, old cloths and rags, mattress pieces, used socks, and grass from the yard) occurs in lower socioeconomic classes in less developed countries, these traditional practices may continue in the families of young women who migrate to a developed country.[8]

In the United States and other high-income countries, clinicians must work to improve awareness of menarche, menstrual hygiene management, and customs regarding reproductive health to better serve patients, particularly those who are recent immigrants from resource-poor countries. Importantly, inadequate education, knowledge, and beliefs about menstrual hygiene management may also be present in the poorest parts of affluent countries. Access to menstrual supplies may be taken for granted and issues obtaining supplies easily overlooked.[8] For example, a white female patient living in a women's shelter with her newborn infant in central Pennsylvania used urine-soiled diapers instead of menstrual pads for her postpartum bleeding because of lack of access to commercial sanitary products.[8] Knowledge and awareness of menarche and menstruation significantly improve through office-based and public health education.[10]

CONTRACEPTION AND FAMILY PLANNING

Contraception use and family planning practices differ greatly. To adequately address contraception availability and promote shared decision making regarding family planning, clinicians should be aware of prior knowledge and use of contraception. Studies show that Syrian refugees in Jordan are widely aware of modern contraceptive methods, including condoms, oral contraception, long-acting reversible contraception, and injectable hormonal contraceptives.[10,11] Eritrean refugees in Ethiopia knew of at least 1 type of modern contraceptive, but less than half had received information about long-term contraception or permanent contraception. Several barriers at the patient, clinician, and system levels affect women's knowledge of, access to, and use of contraceptive methods before arrival. There are significant unmet contraceptive needs among these groups, quantified as the number of women who desire to avoid pregnancy but are not using a modern contraceptive method. Even following settlement in North America, these unmet needs are disproportionately higher than those of nonimmigrant and nonrefugee women.[12]

Before arrival, the main barriers to adequate provision of contraception and counseling on family planning that have been identified are:

1. Inadequate resources, including remote delivery sites, unavailability of some or all options, prohibitive costs
2. Clinician biases for or against certain methods or based on their own cultural beliefs or health practices
3. Lack of or incomplete clinician training
4. Prior trauma, including sex-based and gender-based violence as well as coercive or forced contraception or sterilization

Significant efforts have been made to overcome these barriers in refugee settings, because "the use of contraception can prevent unintended pregnancy, reduce abortion, increase opportunities to attain higher education, and stimulate economic growth."[13]

Clinicians must consider the barriers experienced by immigrant and refugee women in order to deliver a holistic approach to contraceptive care. Start by asking about knowledge and experience with contraception in the past. Ask open-ended questions to determine each patient's goals for family planning. Consider having this conversation with the patient by herself and, if needed, involve an interpreter with whom the patient is comfortable; female interpreters are often preferred. Take care to avoid language or vocabulary that could be interpreted as coercive. Resources are available in a variety of languages, but ensure that the resources cover the complete range of options. Provide each patient with a free, full, and informed choice.

MATERNITY CARE
Prenatal Care

Prenatal care is invaluable; its absence increases not only health care costs but also the morbidity and mortality of the mother and her infant.[14] In the United States, refugee women may arrive at the time of delivery with significant comorbid conditions, the severity of which could have been mitigated by adequate prenatal care. Explanations for this lack of care are multifaceted and include difficulty with navigating a new health care system, decreased knowledge and awareness of services, challenges with gaining cultural acceptance, and health and financial literacy. These difficulties are compounded by limited English proficiency, which causes a sense of loss of autonomy for the patient.[15]

Screening During Pregnancy

Effective screening during prenatal care requires knowledge of specific refugee and immigrant risk factors. To effectively screen, clinicians must familiarize themselves with the unique challenges faced by refugees. Further screening recommendations during pregnancy are provided in **Table 2**.

Beliefs About Delivery

Inherent to the care provided to refugee women is the ability to explore, with care, knowledge and attitudes around delivery. Clinicians should take the time to understand what beliefs and cultural practices are around birth practices. Care should be taken to respect those beliefs. Included in these practices is often a preference for female clinicians during labor and delivery.

Ethnicity and geographic origins have specific risk factors for labor and delivery. Women from sub-Saharan Africa are at higher risk of eclampsia followed by uterine rupture, with a positive correlation noted between eclampsia and number of months since immigration.[16] Hispanic and Caribbean women are at an increased risk of preeclampsia with severe features.[17] There is conflicting evidence for risk of cesarean

Table 2
Screening tests and associated outcomes for pregnant women

Screening	Associated Outcomes	Trimester	Comments
Sexually transmitted infections (human immunodeficiency virus, syphilis, hepatitis B, gonorrhea, and chlamydia)	Preterm birth, stillbirth, neonatal death, low birth weight, sepsis, pneumonia, neonatal conjunctivitis, and congenital deformities	First and third	—
Folate (CBC)	NTDs and cleft palate	First	Supplement 3 mo before conception; 50% decrease in NTD[14]
Anemia (CBC)	Low birth weight, preterm delivery, postpartum hemorrhage, sepsis, postpartum depression	First	Women may have migrated from countries where their iron intake is 50% lower than that of men[16]
Rubella (rubella immunoglobulin G)	Congenital rubella syndrome, fetal demise	First	Lowest vaccine rate in women from North Africa, Middle East, China, and South Pacific[17]
Depression (Edinburgh Postpartum Depression Scale)	Postpartum blues, depression, psychosis	First, third, and fourth	—
Intimate partner violence (Hurt, Insult, Threaten, Scream tool)	Depression, physical violence, child abuse	First, third, and fourth	—
Genetic variant carrier (serum biochemistry, nuchal translucency, hemoglobin electrophoresis)	Congenital disorders, fetal demise, neonatal death	Preconception and second	—

Abbreviations: CBC, complete blood count; NTD, neural tube defect.

delivery and preterm birth; however, recent migration has been found to be a risk factor for low birth weight.

Postpartum

The postpartum period represents a time of increased vulnerability because there is heightened stress and increased reliance on support networks. For many refugee women, establishing a residence in the host country signifies a divorce from their former support networks. Clinicians should identify this risk as early as possible in the course of prenatal care. Connect the patient to support systems by way of local refugee programs, doulas, and peer support groups to help mitigate the isolation and stress that may be encountered during this period.

Breastfeeding

Despite the World Health Organization recommendations to exclusively breastfeed for at least the first 6 months of life, there is variance in the rates of initiation, exclusivity, and continuation of breastfeeding among women. Often, a predictor of breastfeeding initiation is the belief held by a particular culture about the importance of such practice. The longer a patient has spent in the United States, the less likely she is to breastfeed.[18] Some refugee women believe breastfeeding is the life source to their infants after delivery and an inability to do so can result in development of depression and anxiety.[19]

MENTAL HEALTH

The mental health challenges of women who flee or immigrate to the United States include preexisting mental health conditions, a higher likelihood of experiencing trauma during the migration process, and challenges of settling on arrival.[20] Even on resettling, women tend to have less access to education and language training, health care, vocational training and employment, and other services compared with men.[21] Rates of mental health conditions such as anxiety, posttraumatic stress disorder, and depression are higher among refugees than in the general population.[22–24]

Depression

Kiba is a 66-year-old Bhutanese woman. She has been in the United States for 6 years and fled with her son, daughter-in-law, and grandson by way of a refugee camp. Since arriving, she has had little interaction with her extended family, cares for her grandson, stays at home primarily, and has not developed friendships. She cannot speak English or navigate transportation, and cannot easily contact her family in Bhutan.

Patients such as Kiba are at high risk for depression caused by social isolation, lack of community, and divorce from family in their home country. Screen patients for depression using a validated tool such as the Refugee Health Screener-15 (RHS-15). Encourage language classes, engagement in the community, and other social connections. Discuss the long-term implications of fleeing the country and explore her expectations for social integration into the United States and local communities.

Posttraumatic Stress Disorder

Rima is a 34-year-old woman from Syria who arrived in the United States 12 weeks ago after 3 years in a refugee camp. She is accompanied by her 3 children. Before arrival, her RHS-15 was positive for emotional distress. She is initially hesitant to share specific details; however, she acknowledges a history of intimate partner violence, estrangement from her eldest son, and loss of her 2 brothers in the war. She does not sleep well, has frequent nightmares, and has difficulty concentrating during the day.

Identification of posttraumatic stress disorder (PTSD) is necessary to adequately assist patients in managing symptoms. PTSD is up to 10 times more common among refugees and immigrants than in the general population, and it affects women at higher rates than men.[22,24,25] Most commonly associated with traumatic experiences, PTSD can also be related to acculturation, "the process of integrating into a new culture while also maintaining one's origin culture and identity."[24] Even if a patient has not been exposed to characteristic traumatic experiences, understanding the risk of PTSD in displaced persons is crucial to diagnosis and management.[24]

Somatization

Halima is a 42-year-old woman who fled Somalia 4 years ago with her husband and 4 children. She now has 6 children. Since arrival, she has been seen by 1 clinician, and has experienced intermittent abdominal pain. The pain is not characteristic of a specific disorder and she has undergone an extensive evaluation. She completed a course of therapy for the only positive result, *Helicobacter pylori*, 2 years ago.

Somatic symptom disorder is characterized by 1 or more somatic symptoms that are accompanied by excessive thoughts, feelings, and/or behaviors related to the somatic symptoms. The prevalence of somatization varies but it is noted to be significantly higher in non-Western patients than in Western patients.[25–27] Cognitive behavior therapy or referral to a psychologist to review strategies for coping with pain is recommended. Encourage language and vocational training. Clinicians should avoid stereotyping and generalizations to prevent overlooking a serious condition.[27] A multifaceted approach may be necessary, using community resources and community members where appropriate.[20]

TRADITIONAL PRACTICES

Around the world, communities pass down traditions for generations. Although these traditions often unify and celebrate a community's identity, some practices are harmful. In addition to fertility control and birth practices, discussed previously, refugee and immigrant women may be subject to the traditional practices discussed next. It is important for clinicians to be aware of practices that physically harm women and may emotionally harm them.

Female Genital Mutilation

Nearly 200 million women alive have undergone FGM, primarily those from African countries but also those from the Middle East and Asia. FGM typically occurs before the age of 15 years. Ethnicity is the strongest predictor of FGM.[28] Ethnicities highly associated with FGM include Peulh, Kissi, Soussou, and Malinke (Guinea), as well as Bobo, Dioula, Sénoufo, Gourmantché, and Felfudé/Peul Mossi (Burkina Faso).[29] **Table 3** reviews the classification of FGM.

FGM may cause complications during childbirth; formation of cysts, abscesses, or keloid scars; urinary incontinence or urethral damage; dyspareunia; sexual dysfunction; hypersensitivity of genitals; increased risk of human immunodeficiency virus; and psychological ramifications. Infibulation obstructs the vaginal canal. Before intercourse, in many cultures, women are physically cut to enable penetration. However, the space on the vaginal introitus is often not adequate for vaginal delivery, and women are at higher risk for cesarean section and postpartum hemorrhage.[30,31] Infibulation may also result in menstrual disorders, recurring infections, fistulae, and

religious-minorities-are-christians/ft_17-02-03_refugeereligion_640px/. Accessed May 16, 2020.

5. Gagnon AJ, Merry L, Robinson C. A systematic review of refugee women's reproductive health. Refuge Can J Refug 2002;21(1):6–17.

6. World Health Organization. Breast cancer: prevention and control. Cancer. 2020. Available at: http://www.who.int/cancer/detection/breastcancer/en/. Accessed August 2, 2020.

7. National Association of Community Health Centers. PRAPARE. NACHC. 2020. Available at: https://www.nachc.org/research-and-data/prapare/. Accessed May 26, 2020.

8. Kuhlmann AS, Henry K, Wall LL. Menstrual hygiene management in resource-poor countries. Obstet Gynecol Surv 2017;72(6):356–76.

9. Mahon T. Menstrual hygiene in South Asia: a neglected issue for WASH (water, sanitation and hygiene) programmes. Gend Dev 2010;18(1):99–113.

10. Sumpter C, Torondel B. A systematic review of the health and social effects of menstrual hygiene management. PLoS One 2013;8(4):e62004.

11. West L, Isotta-Day H, Ba-Break M, et al. Factors in use of family planning services by Syrian women in a refugee camp in Jordan. J Fam Plann Reprod Health Care 2016;73(2):96–102.

12. Wiebe E. Contraceptive practices and attitudes among immigrant and nonimmigrant women in Canada. Can Fam Physician 2013;59(10):e451–5.

13. Aptekman M, Rashid M, Wright V, et al. Unmet contraceptive needs among refugees. Can Fam Physician Med Fam Can 2014;60(12):e613–9.

14. Outcomes I of M (US) C on IB, Bale JR, Stoll BJ, Lucas AO. Reducing Maternal Mortality and Morbidity. National Academies Press (US). 2003. Available at: https://www.ncbi.nlm.nih.gov/books/NBK222105/. Accessed August 3, 2020.

15. Wikberg A, Bondas T. A patient perspective in research on intercultural caring in maternity care: a meta-ethnography. Int J Qual Stud Health Well-being 2010;5(1). https://doi.org/10.3402/qhw.v5i1.4648.

16. Wilson-Mitchell K, Rummens JA. Perinatal outcomes of uninsured immigrant, refugee and migrant mothers and newborns living in Toronto, Canada. Int J Environ Res Public Health 2013;10(6):2198–213.

17. Urquia ML, Wanigaratne S, Ray JG, et al. Severe maternal morbidity associated with maternal birthplace: a population-based register study. J Obstet Gynaecol Can 2017;39(11):978–87.

18. General (US) O of the S, Prevention (US) C for DC and, Health (US) O on W. Barriers to Breastfeeding in the United States. Office of the Surgeon General (US). 2011. Available at: https://www.ncbi.nlm.nih.gov/books/NBK52688/. Accessed August 3, 2020.

19. Fellmeth G, Fazel M, Plugge E. Migration and perinatal mental health in women from low- and middle-income countries: a systematic review and meta-analysis. BJOG Int J Obstet Gynaecol 2017;124(5):742–52.

20. Herrman H. Sustainable development goals and the mental health of resettled refugee women: a role for international organizations. Front Psychiatry 2019;10. https://doi.org/10.3389/fpsyt.2019.00608.

21. Fisher J, Herrman H, de Mello MC, et al. Women's Mental Health. Oxford University Press. Available at: https://oxfordmedicine.com/view/10.1093/med/9780199920181.001.0001/med-9780199920181-chapter-16. Accessed May 16, 2020.

22. Bogic M, Njoku A, Priebe S. Long-term mental health of war-refugees: a systematic literature review. BMC Int Health Hum Rights 2015;15. https://doi.org/10.1186/s12914-015-0064-9.

23. Anderson FM, Hatch SL, Comacchio C, et al. Prevalence and risk of mental disorders in the perinatal period among migrant women: a systematic review and meta-analysis. Arch Womens Ment Health 2017;20(3):449–62.

24. Hameed S, Sadiq A, Din AU. The increased vulnerability of refugee population to mental health disorders. Kans J Med 2018;11(1):20–3.

25. Adel FW, Bernstein E, Tcheyan M, et al. San Antonio refugees: Their demographics, healthcare profiles, and how to better serve them. PLoS One 2019;14(2). https://doi.org/10.1371/journal.pone.0211930.

26. Fazel M, Wheeler J, Danesh J. Prevalence of serious mental disorder in 7000 refugees resettled in western countries: a systematic review. The Lancet 2005;365(9467):1309–14.

27. Rohlof HG, Knipscheer JW, Kleber RJ. Somatization in refugees: a review. Soc Psychiatry Psychiatr Epidemiol 2014;49(11):1793–804.

28. WHO | Female genital mutilation (FGM). WHO. Available at: http://www.who.int/reproductivehealth/topics/fgm/prevalence/en/.

29. Liang M, Loaiza E, Diop N, et al. Demographic Perspectives on Female Genital Mutilation. United Nations Population Fund. Available at: https://sustainabledevelopment.un.org/content/documents/19961027123_UN_Demograhics_v3%20(1).pdf.

30. Banks E, Meirik O, Farley T, et al, WHO Study Group On Female Genital Mutilation And Obstetric Outcome. Female genital mutilation and obstetric outcome: WHO collaborative prospective study in six African countries. Lancet Lond Engl 2006;367(9525):1835–41.

31. Rodriguez MI, Say L, Abdulcadir J, et al. Clinical indications for cesarean delivery among women living with female genital mutilation. Int J Gynaecol Obstet 2017;139(1):21–7.

32. United Nations Population Fund. Female genital mutilation (FGM) frequently asked questions. Available at: http://resources/female-genital-mutilation-fgm-frequently-asked-questions.

33. Ouldzeidoune N, Keating J, Bertrand J, et al. A description of female genital mutilation and force-feeding practices in Mauritania: implications for the protection of child rights and health. PLoS One 2013;8(4):e60594.

34. Rguibi M. Fattening practices among Moroccan Saharawi women. East Mediterr Health J 2006;12(5):619–24.

35. United Nations Childrens Fund. Ending Child Marriage: Progress and Prospects. UNICEF. 2014. Available at: https://www.unicef.org/media/files/Child_Marriage_Report_7_17_LR..pdf.

36. World Health Organization. World Report on Violence and Health. WHO. 2014. Available at: https://www.who.int/violence_injury_prevention/violence/world_report/en/.

37. Preventing gender-biased sex selection: an interagency statement OHCHR, UNFPA, UNICEF, UN women and WHO. Geneva, Switzerland: World Health Organization (WHO); 2011. Available at: https://apps.who.int/iris/bitstream/handle/10665/44577/9789241501460_eng.pdf.

Mental Health and Illness

Kim S. Griswold, MD, MPH[a],*, Dianne M. Loomis, DNP, FNP-BC[b,1],
Patricia A. Pastore, MSN, FNP-BC[c]

KEYWORDS

- Mental health • Refugee • Asylum seeker • Immigrant • Resilience
- Trauma-informed care • Cultural context

KEY POINTS

- Primary care providers most often are the de facto providers of mental health care for refugees and immigrants.
- Mental health problems may present through somatic health expressions.
- Approaches to mental health and well-being can be achieved with explicit attention to family and cultural contexts and with the use of professional interpreters who have had additional mental health training.
- Optimum care is provided through a trauma-informed approach, emphasizing resilience and built on trusting relationships.

INTRODUCTION

It is the obligation of every person born in a safer room to open the door when someone in danger knocks.[1]

Voluntary migrants (immigrants) and populations forced to flee from home (refugees and asylum seekers) have been subjected to various stressors during their respective migrations. An important distinction is that refugees and asylum seekers most often have witnessed or been subjected to violence, trauma, loss of loved ones, and persecution due to gender, race/ethnicity, religion, or other personal characteristics. Differences in terminology and definitions of migrating populations make evidence-based guidelines and comparisons difficult. Different terms and definitions pose challenges in describing the epidemiology of mental health conditions and diagnosis within primary care (PC) settings. These semantic differences also affect achieving culturally relevant care and treatment (**Fig. 1**).[2]

---

[a] Department of Family Medicine, Jacobs School of Medicine and Biomedical Sciences, Buffalo, NY, USA; [b] Emeritus, University at Buffalo, School of Nursing, Buffalo, NY, USA; [c] 77 Goodell St., Buffalo, NY 14203, USA
[1] Present address: 77 Goodell St., Buffalo, NY 14203, USA
* Corresponding author. 77 Goodell St., Buffalo, NY 14203, USA.
E-mail address: griswol@buffalo.edu

Prim Care Clin Office Pract 48 (2021) 131–145
https://doi.org/10.1016/j.pop.2020.09.009
0095-4543/21/© 2020 Elsevier Inc. All rights reserved.

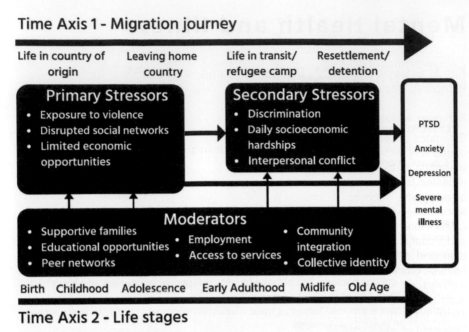

Time Axis 1 - Migration journey

Life in country of origin | Leaving home country | Life in transit/ refugee camp | Resettlement/ detention

Primary Stressors
- Exposure to violence
- Disrupted social networks
- Limited economic opportunities

Secondary Stressors
- Discrimination
- Daily socioeconomic hardships
- Interpersonal conflict

PTSD

Anxiety

Depression

Severe mental illness

Moderators
- Supportive families
- Educational opportunities
- Peer networks
- Employment
- Access to services
- Community integration
- Collective identity

Birth   Childhood   Adolescence   Early Adulthood   Midlife   Old Age

Time Axis 2 - Life stages

Fig. 1. Risk and protective factors for migrant mental health. (*From* Rousseau C, Frounfelker RL. Mental health needs and services for migrants: an overview for primary care providers. J Travel Med 2019;26(2):tay150; with permission.)

BACKGROUND

Our strengths are our power and protect the heart. The power of our strengths will stop hate.[3]

Presentations of mental distress vary enormously because of the heterogeneity of all migrant populations. The severity of mental disorder and responses to management depend on factors that affect all immigrants and refugees: cultural context and beliefs, family circumstances, social supports and social capital, discrimination in the country of resettlement, transnational relationships, and language and literacy.[4]

PREVALENCE OF MENTAL HEALTH PROBLEMS
Immigrants

Of the 44.7 million (13.7%) foreign-born individuals in the United States, Latino and Asian immigrant communities comprise the largest sectors.[5] It has been proposed that as a group, immigrants have lower rates of mental health problems in the early resettlement years, but as time ensues these rates trend toward matching the US-born population.[4,6] This often is referred to as the healthy immigrant effect or immigrant paradox.[4,7] Prevalence studies largely have been completed in refugee populations and thus data in the larger immigrant populations are not known. Overall, the lifetime risk of all psychiatric disorders increases with each generational status (first-generation, second-generation, and third-generation immigrants) due to acculturation.[4,8]

To compare the risk for common mental health problems in immigrants to nonimmigrant populations, it is important to look at the data from a more granular view.

Factors, such as race, ethnicity (and subgroups within each ethnic group), gender, religion, age on immigration, and language proficiency, to name a few, can have an impact on mental health.[4] Caution should be used in drawing broad conclusions of the overall rates of depression, anxiety, substance use disorders, psychotic disorders, and suicidality in this heterogeneous population.

Refugees and Asylum Seekers

Estimates of common mental disorders in adult and children asylum seekers and refugees vary widely; depression from 4% to 62%, anxiety from 4% to 40%, and post-traumatic stress disorder (PTSD) from 8% to 49%.[9] Experiences of torture and repeated trauma are associated strongly with PTSD and depression.[10,11] Conditions of adversity, such as detention, limited access to services, and unemployment, worsen the effects of past trauma.[12,13]

More than half of migrating refugees are children. In contrast to depression (13.81%) and anxiety (15.77%), high rates of PTSD (22.71%) may be found among refugee children and adolescents.[14] Childhood mental disorders may form the backdrop of adverse childhood experiences posing attendant risks to refugee children who have suffered or witnessed traumatic events[15] Country-specific immigration policies, such as family separation, are compounding childhood and familial trauma. This is illustrated by the Physicians for Human Rights (PHR) finding that the US government's treatment of asylum seekers through its policy of family separation constitutes cruel, inhuman, and degrading treatment and, in all cases evaluated by PHR experts, rises to the level of torture.[16]

A high proportion of refugee women flee from gender-based violence in their home countries or encounter rape or other sexual trauma during their journey to presumed safety.[17] Pregnant refugee women may experience a higher rate of postnatal depression, in contrast to native-born women.[18] Like studies focused on nonrefugee populations, risk factors for pregnant refugee women include a prior history of depression, isolation, and poor social supports. There are few data on the prevalence of other mental health problems, such as psychosis.[19,20]

Expressions of psychological distress and psychiatric disorder among lesbian, gay, bisexual, transgender, and queer or questioning asylum-seeking populations may present as somatization, PTSD, or depression and often reflect the persecution suffered in their home countries and repeated traumas.[21] Furthermore, there may be a high incidence of sexual violence and suicidal behaviors.[22]

A recent review looking at suicidal risk among immigrants and ethnic minorities found that overall these groups may be at moderate to high risk of suicidal behavior; notably, risks included separation from family in their home country and language difficulties whereas possible triggers related more to acculturation, loss of social capital and connection, and lack of knowledge of health care systems.[23]

Prevalence of psychotic disorders, such as schizophrenia, schizoaffective disorder, delusional disorders, and bipolar and other psychotic disorders, has been found to be 2%, which is similar to the rate in the general population of the host country.[24]

Substance abuse among refugees, asylum seekers, and irregular migrants are found to be lower immediately after migration; however, they become similar to the host country population over time.[25]

Substance use and abuse may be comorbid with other mental health problems. Screening and management of substance use problems should be undertaken through a cultural lens, ensuring that behavioral health (BH) treatment options are available and accessible.[26,27]

given the cultural background, social circumstances, historical context, and the individual or family's explanatory model of illness.[6,44,50,51] The *Diagnostic and Statistical Manual of Mental Disorders* (Fifth Edition) (*DSM-5*) provides a Cultural Formulation Interview that offers a framework for inquiry during a mental health encounter. The assessment seeks to determine cultural identity of an individual, cultural conceptualizations of distress or suffering, cultural features of vulnerability and resilience, and psychosocial stressors.[52] Common mental health conditions and diagnostic and therapeutic considerations seen in refugees and immigrants are summarized in **Table 2**.

Diagnostic Concepts

Cultural beliefs about mental health vary among heterogeneous groups and may affect their willingness to seek treatment. A majority of patients who experience distress and suffering, however, access PC; hence, PC clinics become out of necessity integrated primary/BH settings.[6] It is helpful to provide education for patients to enhance mental health literacy around psychiatric diagnose and make use of the Cultural Formulation Interview in the *DSM-5*.[6,44] Employ standard evidence-based diagnostic criteria for the conditions most likely to present: PTSD, depression/anxiety, and somatization disorders, keeping in mind conditions may overlap. Remember that somatic symptoms are very real for patients experiencing them. These symptoms should be acknowledged, while at the same time assessing for underlying psychological issues.

When assessing children's mental health, there is evidence that PTSD in refugees may be related to punitive parenting styles, reinforcing the importance of whole-family evaluation and treatment.[53] Always have an index of suspicion for more serious mental illness, such as schizophrenia or psychosis secondary to major depression. Be mindful of cultural expressions and stigma within cultural groups and wider society, and remain alert particularly to the possibility of suicidal thinking or intent.[23,54]

Treatment Approaches

Educate and train all providers in the appropriate use of interpreters and in transcultural, trauma-informed care.[31,55,56] If patients present with prior diagnoses of serious mental illness, clinicians may prescribe bridging psychotropic medications while making appropriate referrals, if necessary. Few studies address the ethnopharmacologic effect of psychotherapeutic agents in diverse populations, and the overall pharmacokinetic effects are unclear in heterogeneous populations.[57] In addition, the environment, cultural dietary practices, and medicinal herbal remedies can have an impact on drug response.[58,59] For at-risk populations, it is suggested to start low and to increase slowly.

Trauma-informed practices focus on resiliency and build trust. Trauma-informed providers ask for permission when approaching difficult issues and recognize current factors in the person's life that may compound suffering.[46,60,61] Family interventions for refugees and immigrants are critically important in addressing the aftermath of trauma.[62] With all interactions, ensure that appropriate BH follow-up and treatment are available, if needed, particularly for patients with psychotic disorders or with suicidal ideation or intent.

Innovations in Care

Treatment modalities for traumatized refugees that are not practiced uniformly have been described. Seven Recovery-Oriented Survivor Empowerment Strategies focuses on coping resources and self-efficacy and the development of skills to alter negative situations. The WHO Problem Management Plus delivers transdiagnostic (across comorbid conditions) behavioral psychological interventions in low-resource and middle-resource countries, using guided self-help to reduce psychological

Table 2
Mental health evaluation and management for refugees and immigrants

Mental Health Diagnosis	Diagnostic Recommendations	Treatment Considerations
Mental health assessment	• Assess all presentations through a cultural lens, sociohistorical background, and the individual's explanatory model of illness and health. • Utilize the Cultural Formulation Interview of the *DSM-5*, when appropriate. • Hierarchal approach from safety to community strengthening to focused psychosocial interventions and clinical services.[36] • Use medically trained interpreters. • Focus on functional status.[35] • Consider traumatic brain injury, neurologic problems, acute stress, grief, depression, psychosis, PTSD, epilepsy, intellectual disability, substance use disorder, suicide and other conditions that impair functioning.[40] • Be aware that Western models of mental health care may not resonate with individuals from other cultural backgrounds.	• Identify strengths, social supports, and access to appropriate PC services. • Provide education about stress and mental health resources.[37] • DO NO HARM—build on strengths.[36] • Family interventions may be particularly helpful. • Models of care include utilizing a variety of interventions: low-intensity peer-led mental health support; integrated care; and use of high-quality interpreters and cultural mediators to improve engagement in health services.[38] • Focus on education to enhance mental health literacy. • Ensure appropriate and timely follow-up. • If using pharmacotherapy, remember that cultural dietary practice and use of medicinal herbs may affect pharmacokinetics. • Provides pharmacologic and psychosocial interventions for adults and for special populations (children, adolescents, and pregnant or breastfeeding and older adults).[41]
Major depressive disorder	• Screen for depression using interpreters for clinical interviews (provider language discordant) or use of linguistically concordant screening tools (caution with cultural validity of tools) only when coordinated systems are in place.[37,39] • Depression screening tools-must be translated into appropriate language (Primary Care Evaluation of Mental Health Disorders, Patient Health Questionnair-9, depression section of Hopkins Symptom Checklist).[37]	• Treatment of depression involves stepped care approaches, psychoeducation, pharmacotherapy, culturally tailored counselling, and follow-up.[39]

(continued on next page)

Table 2
(continued)

Mental Health Diagnosis	Diagnostic Recommendations	Treatment Considerations
PTSD	• No routine screening about trauma; caution about probing about trauma in well-functioning individuals.[39]	• Spontaneous recovery from traumatic events can occur once safety is achieved (80% individuals).[39] • Practice trauma-informed care, build trust and acknowledge resiliency. • PTSD interventions include NET and trauma-focused cognitive behavior therapy.[38]
Psychotic disorders	• Acute psychiatric or severe chronic mental health problems with severe functional impairment require immediate evaluation and may need referral. • With chronic psychiatric conditions where functional impairment is present, but no harm to self or others, facilitate linkage to mental health services or integrated care.	• Pharmacologic and psychosocial interventions for adults and for special populations (children, adolescents, and pregnant or breastfeeding and older adults).[41]
Somatization	• Suspect ongoing trauma-related problems in individuals with somatic complaints, depression, anxiety, and insomnia.[39]	• Acknowledge somatic symptoms while remaining alert to underlying psychosocial or psychological issues.

distress. Another innovation that warrants attention is narrative exposure therapy (NET), which examines trauma as part of the entire life history of the person.[63–65]

Concepts from front-line PC with refugees include videos with suggestions for promoting wellness and mental health and how trauma affects the mental health of refugee communities.[66,67]

A recent TED Talk explores bringing mental health services to refugees in camps, reframing traumatic experiences in order to mitigate long-term or cumulative trauma.[68]

Resilience and resistance are formidable qualities of immigrants and refugees. Strength, adaptability, purpose, hopefulness, and flexibility are attributes that mitigate poor psychological responses. Protective factors include social networks and community stability.[65] Providers can educate themselves and their clinical teams about the important contributions of family connections and transnational linkages to resilience and well-being.[4,50]

CULTURALLY INFORMED MODEL OF CARE

Refugee patients can strengthen physicians' own resilience, another timely topic in this era of burnout. Working with refugees can reinvigorate a sense of purpose among clinicians.[54]

This article draws from more than 20 years of collaboration between the authors in a family medicine practice with a large immigrant/refugee population. As novice PC providers and an expanding practice with the influx of several cultures, the authors began innovative process improvements, adding refugee health to monthly staff meetings and placing pictures of providers with names and titles in the lobby and signage in the clinic translated into languages representing the community. Medically trained interpreters and telephonic interpretation were utilized. A welcome health brochure was written and translated on what to expect at the PC appointments. A prayer room was requested and opened for Arabic Muslim patients for Salah. Staff were hired representing the refugee community. Through local university affiliations, the authors trained medical students, registered nurses (RNs), and nurse practitioner (NP) students to provide clinical experiences and cultural training with the hopes that this experience would develop culturally competent practitioners. Partnerships between refugee resettlement agencies forged a collaboration between patients and other medical providers in the surrounding community. Funding was received through American Academy of Family Physicians Research Stimulation Grant Program for those with severe mental health illness who attended an assertive community treatment program, which included refugees. A behavioral health liaison and a psychiatric care basic tool kit were practice enhancements that were shown to be helpful in accessing and navigating PC.[69]

Listening to their voices while also assessing the physical and psychosocial needs of multigenerational families led to an integrated PC and BH clinic using the collaborative care model. Embedded PC with BH included psychiatrists, psychiatric NPs, RNs and care managers, pharmacists, and peer support for those with mental health disorders, including serious mental illness and addictions. This included culturally informed comprehensive transitional care from inpatient to outpatient settings, family support, and referrals to community and social support services. The experiences strengthened the providers' own resilience and resolve. Looking back at the progress made and seeing patients succeed in the community continue to be invigorating. Hearing refugees' stories challenged providers to work better as a team. Utilizing data from quality improvement projects, the environment and workflow were redesigned to improve efficiencies and transitioned to a more culturally informed practice.[70]

SUMMARY AND FUTURE DIRECTIONS

Through the world of The United Nations Health Commissioner for Refugees (UNHCR)...we witness the courage, tenacity and brilliance of refugees every single day...Striving to belong, and to contribute, they reach out to their new neighbors, building connections, and creating new opportunities.[71]

PC providers can utilize many strategies to promote mental well-being and focus on resilience and the social determinants of health. Often missing in the literature are the voices of refugees and immigrants themselves. Integrated or collaborative care models are ideal for delivering optimum care for refugee and immigrant communities. Connecting primary and behavioral care promotes a team approach; provides comprehensive, whole-person care; and, most importantly, relies on the participation of patients and families in their care.[72] Integrated care is efficacious for trauma and torture survivors and has proved valuable in work with refugee children and with populations of limited English proficiency.[73–76] Utilizing collaborative care models offers opportunities to address social determinants of health in communities and establish "sustainable changes in the health care system."[77]

CLINICS CARE POINTS

- When caring for refugees, consider distinctive family circumstances, social support and social capital, cultural discrimination in resettlement, and language and literacy.
- Resilience is dependent on the unique dynamics of the individual, family, and community.
- Before conducting a physical examination or discussing invasive diagnostic testing, it is crucial to begin sensitive inquiry about torture history.
- Refugees and asylum seekers may present with somatic concerns, insomnia, and PTSD that may be reflective of torture.
- To decrease stigma and improve access rates to PC and mental health services, form specific action plans for community outreach.
- Practice cultural humility and the skill of being a "learner" as a provider to mitigate perceived discrimination on the part of the patient. Be advocates in and for refugee and immigrant communities.
- It is important to discover key similarities and differences among immigrant populations. Providers and researchers can be guided by the social determinants of health.
- The complex postmigration milieu may have profound influence on refugee children and adolescents. Providers need to focus interventions toward parents and the social determinants of health. School-based initiatives have a crucial role.

DISCLOSURE

The Authors have nothing to disclose.

REFERENCES

1. Nayeri D. The ungrateful refugee: 'We have no debt to repay'. 2017. Available at: https://www.theguardian.com/world/2017/apr/04/dina-nayeri-ungrateful-refugee. [Accessed 6 May 2020].

2. Rousseau C, Frounfelker RL. Mental health needs and services for migrants: an overview for primary care providers. J Trav Med 2019;26(2).
3. Fabio M, Parker LD, Siddharth MB. Building on resiliencies of refugee families. Pediatr Clin North Am 2019;66(3):655–67.
4. Alegria M, Alvarez K, DiMarzio K. Immigration and mental health. Curr Epidemiol Rep 2017;4(2):145–55.
5. Foreign born: selected characteristics of the foreign-born population by period of entry into the United States American Community Survey [website]. 2018. Available at: https://data.census.gov/cedsci/table?q=Foreign%20Born&hidePreview=false&t=Foreign%20Born&tid=ACSST1Y2018.S0502&vintage=2018. [Accessed 6 May 2020].
6. Kirmayer LJ, Narasiah L, Munoz M, et al. Common mental health problems in immigrants and refugees: general approach in primary care. CMAJ 2011;183(12): E959–67.
7. Durbin A, Moineddin R, Lin E, et al. Mental health service use by recent immigrants from different world regions and by non-immigrants in Ontario, Canada: a cross-sectional study. BMC Health Serv Res 2015;15:336.
8. Shekunov J. Immigration and risk of psychiatric disorders: a review of existing literature. Am J Psychiatry Resid J 2016;11(2):3–5.
9. Turrini G, Purgato M, Ballette F, et al. Common mental disorders in asylum seekers and refugees: umbrella review of prevalence and intervention studies. Int J Ment Health Syst 2017;11(1):51.
10. Silove D, Ventevogel P, Rees S. The contemporary refugee crisis: an overview of mental health challenges. World Psychiatry 2017;16(2):130–9.
11. Shawyer F, Enticott JC, Block AA, et al. The mental health status of refugees and asylum seekers attending a refugee health clinic including comparisons with a matched sample of Australian-born residents. BMC Psychiatry 2017;17(1):76.
12. Steel Z, Chey T, Silove D, et al. Association of torture and other potentially traumatic events with mental health outcomes among populations exposed to mass conflict and displacement: a systematic review and meta-analysis. JAMA 2009;302(5):537–49.
13. Steel Z, Silove D, Brooks R, et al. Impact of immigration detention and temporary protection on the mental health of refugees. Br J Psychiatry 2006;188:58–64.
14. Blackmore R, Gray KM, Boyle JA, et al. Systematic review and meta-analysis: the prevalence of mental illness in child and adolescent refugees and asylum seekers. J Am Acad Child Adolesc Psychiatry 2019;59(6):705–14.
15. Liu M. War and children. Am J Psychiatry Resid J 2017;12(7):3–5.
16. Habbach H, Hampton K, Mishori R. "You will never see your child again" The persistent psychological effects of family separation [website]. 2020. Available at: https://phr.org/our-work/resources/you-will-never-see-your-child-again-the-persistent-psychological-effects-of-family-separation/. [Accessed 6 May 2020].
17. Parish A. Gender-based violence against women: both cause for migration and risk along the journey. [website]. 2017. Available at: https://www.migrationpolicy.org/article/gender-based-violence-against-women-both-cause-migration-and-risk-along-journey. Accessed May 7, 2020.
18. Collins CH, Zimmerman C, Howard LM. Refugee, asylum seeker, immigrant women and postnatal depression: rates and risk factors. Arch Womens Ment Health 2011;14(1):3–11.
19. Fellmeth G, Fazel M, Plugge E. Migration and perinatal mental health in women from low- and middle-income countries: a systematic review and meta-analysis. BJOG 2017;124(5):742–52.

20. Johnson-Agbakwu CE, Allen J, Nizigiyimana JF, et al. Mental health screening among newly arrived refugees seeking routine obstetric and gynecologic care. Psychol Serv 2014;11(4):470–6.
21. Messih M. Mental health in LGBT refugee populations. Am J Psychiatry Resid J 2016;11(7):5–7.
22. Hopkinson RA, Keatley E, Glaeser E, et al. Persecution experiences and mental health of LGBT asylum seekers. J Homosex 2017;64(12):1650–66.
23. Forte A, Trobia F, Gualtieri F, et al. Suicide risk among immigrants and ethnic minorities: a literature overview. Int J Environ Res Public Health 2018;15(7).
24. World at war. UN Refugee Agency; 2014. Available at: https://www.unhcr.org/en-us/statistics/country/556725e69/unhcr-global-trends-2014.html Accessed October 21, 2020.
25. Teunissen E, van den Bosch L, van Bavel E, et al. Mental health problems in undocumented and documented migrants: a survey study. Fam Pract 2014;31(5):571–7.
26. Horyniak D, Melo JS, Farrell RM, et al. Epidemiology of substance use among forced migrants: a global systematic review. PLoS One 2016;11(7):e0159134.
27. Posselt M, Galletly C, de Crespigny C, et al. Mental health and drug and alcohol comorbidity in young people of refugee background: a review of the literature. Ment Health Subst Use 2014;7(1):19–30.
28. Fox M, Thayer ZM, Wadhwa PD. Acculturation and health: the moderating role of sociocultural context. Am Anthropol 2017;119(3):405–21.
29. Derr AS. Mental health service use among immigrants in the United States: a systematic review. Psychiatr Serv 2016;67(3):265–74.
30. Bauldry S, Szaflarski M. Immigrant-based disparities in mental health care utilization. Socius 2017;3.
31. Wylie L, Van Meyel R, Harder H, et al. Assessing trauma in a transcultural context: challenges in mental health care with immigrants and refugees. Public Health Rev 2018;39:22.
32. Bartolomei J, Baeriswyl-Cottin R, Framorando D, et al. What are the barriers to access to mental healthcare and the primary needs of asylum seekers? A survey of mental health caregivers and primary care workers. BMC Psychiatry 2016;16(1):336.
33. Chiarenza A, Dauvrin M, Chiesa V, et al. Supporting access to healthcare for refugees and migrants in European countries under particular migratory pressure. BMC Health Serv Res 2019;19(1):513.
34. Brisset C, Leanza Y, Rosenberg E, et al. Language barriers in mental health care: a survey of primary care practitioners. J Immigr Minor Health 2014;16(6):1238–46.
35. Singleton G, Hocking D, Gardiner J, et al. Mental health. In: Norberry D, editor. Recommendations for comprehensive post-arrival health assessment for people from refugee-like backgrounds. 2nd edition. Surry Hills (NSW): Australasian Society for Infectious Diseases; 2016. p. 141–7.
36. Operational guidance mental health & psychosocial support programming for refugee operations. Geneva: United Nations High Commissioner for Refugees (UNCHR); 2013.
37. U.S. Department of Health and Human Services Centers for Disease Control and Prevention National Center for Emerging and Zoonotic Infectious Diseases Division of Global Migration and Quaratine. Guidelines for mental health screening during the domestic medical examination for newly arrived refugees 2015.

Available at: https://www.cdc.gov/immigrantrefugeehealth/guidelines/domestic/mental-health-screening-guidelines.html Accessed October 21, 2020.

38. Mental health promotion and mental health care in refugees and migrants: technical guidance. Copenhagen: WHO Regional Office for Europe; 2018.

39. Pottie K, Greenaway C, Feightner J, et al. Evidence-based clinical guidelines for immigrants and refugees. CMAJ 2011;183(12):E824–925.

40. mhGAP humanitarian intervention guide (mhGAP-HIG): clinical management of mental, neurological and substance use conditions in humanitarian emergencies. Geneva: World Health Organization (WHO); 2015.

41. mhGAP intervention guide mental health gap action programme version 2.0 for mental, neurological and substance use disorders in non-specialized health settings. Geneva: World Health Organization (WHO); 2016.

42. mhGAP operations manual: mental health Gap Action Programme (mhGAP). Geneva: World Health Organization; 2018.

43. van den Muijsenbergh M. Migrant mental health care. In: Dowrick C, editor. Global primary mental health care: practical guidance for family doctors. London: Routledge; 2019. p. 91.

44. Kronick R. Mental health of refugees and asylum seekers: assessment and intervention. Can J Psychiatry 2018;63(5):290–6.

45. Shannon PJ, Vinson GA, Wieling E, et al. Torture, war trauma, and mental health symptoms of newly arrived Karen refugees. J Loss Trauma 2015;20(6):577–90.

46. Novick DR. Sit back and Listen — the relevance of ptients' stories to trauma-informed care. N Engl J Med 2018;379(22):2093–4.

47. Kleinman A, Eisenberg L, Good B. Culture, illness, and care: clinical lessons from anthropologic and cross-cultural research. Ann Intern Med 1978;88(2):251–8.

48. Lin EH, Carter WB, Kleinman AM. An exploration of somatization among Asian refugees and immigrants in primary care. Am J Public Health 1985;75(9):1080–4.

49. Lanzara R, Scipioni M, Conti C. A clinical-psychological perspective on somatization among immigrants: a systematic review. Front Psychol 2019;9(2792).

50. Mann C, Fazil Q. Mental illness in asylum seekers and refugees. Prim Care Ment Health 2006;4:57–66.

51. Pottie K, Martin JP, Cornish S, et al. Access to healthcare for the most vulnerable migrants: a humanitarian crisis. Confl Health 2015;9(1):16.

52. Cultural formulation. 5th edition. Arlington (VA): American Psychiatric Association; 2013.

53. Bryant RA, Edwards B, Creamer M, et al. The effect of post-traumatic stress disorder on refugees' parenting and their children's mental health: a cohort study. Lancet Public Health 2018;3(5):e249–58.

54. Walden J. Refugee mental health: a primary care approach. Am Fam Physician 2017;96(2):81–4.

55. Kirmayer LJ, Groleau D, Guzder J, et al. Cultural consultation: a model of mental health service for multicultural societies. Can J Psychiatry 2003;48(3):145–53.

56. U.S. Department of Health and Human Services Substance Abuse and Mental Health Services Administration. SAMHSA's concept of trauma and guidance for a trauma-Informed approach. Rockville (MD): HHS Publication; 2014. No. (SMA) 14-4884.

57. Hilgenberg C, Munoz C. Ethnopharmacology. Am J Nurs 2005;105(8):40–9.

58. Lin KM, Smith MW, Ortiz V. Culture and psychopharmacology. Psychiatr Clin North Am 2001;24(3):523–38.

59. Ninnemann KM. Variability in the efficacy of psychopharmaceuticals: contributions from pharmacogenomics, ethnopsychopharmacology, and psychological and psychiatric anthropologies. Cult Med Psychiatry 2012;36(1):10–25.
60. Miller KK, Brown CR, Shramko M, et al. Applying trauma-informed practices to the care of refugee and immigrant youth: 10 clinical pearls. Children 2019;6(8).
61. Bowen EA, Murshid NS. Trauma-informed social policy: a conceptual framework for policy analysis and advocacy. Am J Public Health 2016;106(2):223–9.
62. Caspi Y, Slobodin O, Klein E. Cultural perspectives on the aftereffects of combat trauma: review of a community study of bedouin IDF servicemen and their families. Rambam Maimonides Med J 2015;6(2):e0021.
63. van Heemstra HE, Scholte WF, Haagen JFG, et al. 7ROSES, a transdiagnostic intervention for promoting self-efficacy in traumatized refugees: a first quantitative evaluation. Eur J Psychotraumatol 2019;10(1):1673062.
64. Dawson KS, Bryant RA, Harper M, et al. Problem management plus (PM+): a WHO transdiagnostic psychological intervention for common mental health problems. World Psychiatry 2015;14(3):354–7.
65. Jongedijk RA. Narrative exposure therapy: an evidence-based treatment for multiple and complex trauma. Eur J Psychotraumatol 2014;5:26522.
66. Voices of care: promoting wellness in refugee health - communication [YouTube]. 2014. Available at: https://www.youtube.com/watch?v=sJ5nqghC6l0&feature=youtu.be&list=PLln3-X95CtqSgV2iinsuH3Arc4llX4HFP. [Accessed 20 May 2020].
67. Voices of care: promoting wellness in refugee health - trauma & refugee communities. 2014. Available at: https://youtu.be/S91MyLXFKCl. [Accessed 20 May 2020].
68. Doad E. How we can bring mental health support to refugees. 2018. Available at: https://www.ted.com/talks/essam_daod_how_we_can_bring_mental_health_support_to_refugees?language=en. [Accessed 20 May 2020].
69. Pastore P, Griswold KS, Homish GG, et al. Family practice enhancements for patients with severe mental illness. Community Ment Health J 2013;49(2):172–7.
70. Griswold K, Scates J, Kadhum A. Transforming well-being for refugees and their communities: perspectives from medicine, nursing, education, and social work. In: Smith KH, Ram PK, editors. Transforming global health: interdisciplinary challenges, perspectives, and strategies. Cham: Springer International Publishing; 2020. p. 35–50.
71. Statement by UN High Commissioner for refugees, Filippo Grandi on World Refugee Day 2017. 2017. Available at: https://www.unhcr.org/en-us/news/press/2017/6/5948d2514/statement-un-high-commissioner-refugees-filippo-grandi-world-refugee-day.html. [Accessed 7 May 2020].
72. A quick start guide to behavioral health integration for safety-net primary care providers. Available at: https://www.integration.samhsa.gov/integrated-care-models/CIHS_quickStart_decisiontree_with_links_as.pdf. [Accessed 7 May 2020].
73. Abu Suhaiban H, Grasser LR, Javanbakht A. Mental health of refugees and torture survivors: a critical review of prevalence, predictors, and integrated care. Int J Environ Res Public Health 2019;16(13).
74. Esala JJ, Vukovich MM, Hanbury A, et al. Collaborative care for refugees and torture survivors: Key findings from the literature. Traumatology 2018;24(3):168–85.
75. Rousseau C, Measham T, Nadeau L. Addressing trauma in collaborative mental health care for refugee children. Clin Child Psychol Psychiatry 2012;18(1):121–36.

76. Njeru JW, DeJesus RS, St Sauver J, et al. Utilization of a mental health collaborative care model among patients who require interpreter services. Int J Ment Health Syst 2016;10:15.
77. Bholat MA, Ray L, Brensilver M, et al. Integration of behavioral medicine in primary care. Prim Care 2012;39(4):605–14.
78. Spitzer RL, Kroenke K, Williams JB. Validation and utility of a self-report version of PRIME-MD: the PHQ primary care study. primary care evaluation of mental disorders. Patient health questionnaire. JAMA 1999;282(18):1737–44. Available at: http://www.phqscreeners.com/. Accessed July 13, 2020.
79. Weathers FW, Litz B, Herman D, et al. The PTSD Checklist (PCL): reliability, validity, and diagnostic utility. Volume presented at the Annual Meeting of the International Society for Traumatic Stress Studies; 1993; San Antonio, TX. Available at: https://www.index.va.gov/search/va/va_search.jsp?NQ=URL%3Ahttps%3A%2F%2Fwww.ptsd.va.gov%2Fprofessional%2Fpages%2Fassessments%2Fptsd-checklist.asp&QT=pcl-c&submit.x=0&submit.y=0. Accessed July 13, 2020.
80. Hollifield M, Verbillis-Kolp S, Farmer B, et al. The Refugee Health Screener-15 (RHS-15): development and validation of an instrument for anxiety, depression, and PTSD in refugees. Gen Hosp Psychiatry 2013;35(2):202–9. Available at: https://www.index.va.gov/search/va/va_search.jsp?NQ=URL%3Ahttps%3A%2F%2Fwww.ptsd.va.gov%2Fprofessional%2Fpages%2Fassessments%2Fptsd-checklist.asp&QT=pcl-c&submit.x=0&submit.y=0. Accessed July 13, 2020.
81. Spitzer RL, Kroenke K, Williams JB, et al. A brief measure for assessing generalized anxiety disorder: the GAD-7. Arch Intern Med 2006;166(10):1092–7. Available at: https://www.phqscreeners.com/. Accessed July 13, 2020.
82. Goodman R. The strengths and difficulties questionnaire: a research note. J Child Psychol Psychiatry 1997;38(5):581–6. Available at: http://www.sdqinfo.org/a0.html; http://www.sdqinfo.org/py/sdqinfo/b0.py. Accessed July 13, 2020.
83. Jellinek MS, Murphy JM, Burns BJ. Brief psychosocial screening in outpatient pediatric practice. J Pediatr 1986;109(2):371–8. Available at: https://www.brightfutures.org/mentalhealth/pdf/professionals/ped_sympton_chklst.pdf. Accessed July 13, 2020.
84. Jellinek MS, Murphy JM, Robinson J, et al. Pediatric Symptom Checklist: screening school-age children for psychosocial dysfunction. J Pediatr 1988;112(2):201–9. Available at: https://www.brightfutures.org/mentalhealth/pdf/professionals/ped_sympton_chklst.pdf. Accessed July 13, 2020.

NAVIGATING HEALTH CARE IN THE UNITED STATES
Managing Expectations

> Sarah is an 11-year-old female refugee from the Democratic Republic of the Congo by way of Rwanda who arrived in the US with her parents and 5 siblings. At 5 years old, although living in a refugee camp, Sarah suffered meningitis, which left her quadriplegic and with a seizure disorder. Before her overseas medical examination, Sarah had had no pharmacologic or therapeutic intervention for her condition. On arriving in the US, she was quickly connected to an interdisciplinary primary care clinic and referred to several specialists. Sarah received adaptive equipment, enrolled in school with an Individualized Education Plan, and her seizures were controlled with medication. Sarah's care team was pleased with her progress; however, when a physical therapist asked Sarah's mother about long-term goals for Sarah, she replied, "for her to be able to talk and walk like my other children." The realization that Sarah's parents held unrealistic expectations for Sarah's prognosis informed all future conversations with the family. In subsequent appointments, Sarah's care team celebrated Sarah's progress while providing realistic expectations for Sarah's future level of function. Despite the compassion demonstrated by Sarah's care team, these conversations often resulted in heartache for her parents.

For immigrants from poor or war-torn countries with minimal health care resources, there often exists an idea that the US health care system offers a panacea. Sarah's case highlights the need to discuss expectations early in the treatment of chronic and congenital medical conditions. Assessing the patient's and their family's understanding of their condition, health literacy, and expectations for treatment are vital to building trust and rapport. For those who are able to access Medicaid or private insurance, it may come as a surprise that many services and medications are not covered. Discussing these limitations with patients can prevent surprise medical bills. Kleinman's 8 questions from the Explanatory Model's Approach[1] is a starting point for establishing a common understanding of expectations for health care management, as detailed in by Tan and Allen in their article.

The provision of health care in the US may vary dramatically from what an immigrant has experienced in their country of origin. Some immigrants are accustomed to a paternalistic style of care delivery and may be slow to engage in shared decision-making. Many immigrants come from situations in which they possess little control over their own lives, leading to high expectations for others and a low sense of self-efficacy. Recognizing the strength they have demonstrated in overcoming hardships and tapping to their own resilience is vital for the recovery of self-efficacy.

Health Literacy

> Noele is a 52-year-old woman from Somalia. Shortly on resettlement, she underwent thyroidectomy for a goiter and was placed on levothyroxine. During a follow-up appointment several months later, Noele shared that she was no longer taking the levothyroxine. When asked why she had stopped her medication, Noele explained that where she was from, when you had surgery a problem was fixed, and you did not need to take medication any more. The registered nurse (RN) care coordinator provided education on the location and function of the thyroid gland, using illustrations and finding shared concepts such as the pedals on the car her daughter drives. The patient was able to teach-back the information about the thyroid gland, how to take the medication daily, and how to obtain refills.

The best, most up-to-date health advice is meaningless if it is not understood by the patient. Health literacy is "the degree to which an individual has the capacity to obtain, communicate, process, and understand basic health information and services to make appropriate health decisions."[2] Although some immigrants possess a basic understanding of the functioning of the body, others have no previous experience with concepts such as chronic disease or germ theory. Successful communication begins with eliciting the patient's understanding of their health. The health care provider may need to use creativity to uncover shared concepts that can be used to bridge knowledge gaps, as in the use of car pedals to convey the function of the thyroid gland for Noele. Use of the teach-back method is critical to assess comprehension. The health care provider should invite the patient to ask questions.

Reaching Patients Between Visits

The language barrier is not the only obstacle to communicating with refugee and immigrant patients. Investing a little extra time to reach patients between visits to discuss results, a plan of care, or help navigate referrals and follow-up can result in better care for the patient. Refer to **Table 1** for challenges and helpful hints for connecting with patients.

Table 1	
Challenges and helpful hints for connecting with patients	
Challenges	**Helpful Hints**
• Cellular plans can run out of minutes, leaving the patient unreachable by phone. • Some patients are unlikely to answer the phone from anyone other than a friend who they know will speak their language. • Dialing through a third-party language line may display a number that is mistaken for spam. • Patients may be unaware of how to set up or access voicemail, or their voicemail may be full. • Because of regional variations in language, the patient and interpreter may not understand each other well. • When calling the clinic, the patient may struggle to navigate the call menu. • Automatically generated appointment reminders and other mailed communications are typically printed in English. • Patient portals are typically available only in English.	• Take the time at the initial clinic visit to make sure the patient knows how to call the clinic and request an interpreter. Explain how the clinic will communicate with the patient. • If consent has been documented, consider reaching out to organizations working with the patient (eg, the resettlement agency, community health agency, school, or social services) for updated contact information. • If the patient is not answering a call made through a language service line because they do not recognize the number, try calling from the clinic phone directly; let the patient know you will call right back with an interpreter.

Accessing Care

D.G. is a Kurundi-speaking refugee from the Burundi who recently resettled in the US. At his initial clinic visit, D.G.'s primary care provider notes that he has trouble seeing and would benefit from an eye examination. The university eye clinic is well equipped to offer interpretation services, but D.G.'s managed care Medicaid plan does not cover eye examinations through

In a tight housing market, landlords have little motivation to make property improvements or honor landlord-tenant agreements; renters may be uncomfortable advocating for their rights for fear of retaliatory eviction. Immigrants are in a particularly precarious position of not being familiar with their rights, dealing with a language barrier, and facing discrimination. Housing discrimination is difficult to detect on an individual level, but is nonetheless real. Compared with white renters, Black, Hispanic, and Asian renters are informed of and shown fewer units.[10] In particular, Arab or Muslim applicants are more likely to experience discrimination than other racial or ethnic groups.[11] Medical legal partnerships are invaluable resources for advocating for our immigrant patients.

SCHOOL

More than half of the world's refugees are children,[12] and the past decade has seen an increase in the number of families with children and unaccompanied minors crossing the US-Mexico border in pursuit of asylum.[13] For some immigrants, the public school system may be the first opportunity for a safe education. Voluntary migrants commonly cite education for their children as a reason for immigrating to the US. In addition to the formal curriculum, the social environment of school provides immigrant children with the opportunity to learn the English language and American culture. The education system can be difficult to navigate for immigrant families, especially those with limited English or technology skills.

School Enrollment

School enrollment policies vary from state to state. In some states, each school district has the authority to determine the age cut-off for high school enrollment. Even in a district that allows students to enroll in public school until the age of 21 years, an immigrant arriving in the US at 18 years of age could be denied the opportunity to go to public high school if they arrive without English skills or transcripts from previous schooling, which can be disheartening for families and particularly so for teens who did not attain a high school degree in their home country or country of asylum. Policies for grade placement also vary by district, although students are commonly placed in the grade at or 1 year less than their age at the time of enrollment.

School Physicals and Immunizations

Although refugees will have had many of the necessary vaccines during their overseas medical examination, the same is not true for Special Immigrant Visa holders, Diversity Visa holders, or immigrants who are in the country without authorization. ORR-eligible populations, including refugees and Special Immigrant Visas, can sometimes receive school entrance examinations and immunizations at local health departments. Other populations often rely on low-cost or free clinics to obtain the needed medical verification for school enrollment. Although the CDC provides guidance for a catch-up immunization schedule,[14] providers should defer to their local health department for state-specific vaccine requirements for school enrollment. A best practice is to maintain school examination and vaccination reports in the patient's electronic medical record; this protects the records should the child have delays in enrollment or move across school district lines.

Communication Barriers with Schools

Per joint guidance released by the Departments of Justice and Education, it is the responsibility of schools to provide proper interpretation and translation[15];

unfortunately, this ideal is not always met. Barriers to proper language access include a lack of resources at the school level, staff discomfort in using interpretation, or a misconception that children can serve as interpreters for their parents or guardians. The latter is never appropriate.

School notices are often indecipherable to the parents tasked with reading or signing them. An example of this disconnect is the sixth grade flier informing parents and guardians of the need for the TDaP vaccine before starting seventh grade[16]; some parents and guardians keep their child home from school the next day, believing the communication to mean that the child is forbidden from returning to school until they have received the vaccination.

School Readiness

Immigrant children may arrive in the US with inconsistent school attendance histories. Some school-aged children may have spent their entire lives in refugee camps.[17] Many refugee children receive schooling in camps before resettlement; however, more than half of school-aged refugees have not attended school regularly. Secondary school attendance in camps is particularly dismal, with less than 25% of school-aged refugees attending.[12] Few educators specifically train to work with immigrant students and typically learn that the student is joining their class on the very day the student starts.[18] Immigrants may find it challenging to learn Business English in the classroom and casual vernacular from their peers in the hallways. Immigrants may not have the support needed to stay engaged with schoolwork at home, and teachers struggle to communicate with the parents and guardians of their students with limited English proficiency.

The evaluation to determine a child's supplemental support needs for an Individualized Education Plan is conducted mostly in English. When appropriate testing is not available in a student's language or through nonverbal methods, the student may miss out on necessary support, as their academic problems may be falsely attributed to language deficits. This is particularly troubling due to the high prevalence of adverse childhood experiences in immigrant children.[19] Growing up in war zones, suffering limited resources, and witnessing violence lead to higher than average prevalence of depression, posttraumatic stress disorder, and learning disabilities in immigrant children. Without proper intervention, these children are left behind their peers.

CHANGING FAMILY DYNAMICS

> Hamida is an Afghan Special Immigrant Visa holder who arrived in the US with her husband and 6 children. After she delivered a baby in Afghanistan, her mother and sisters came to her home to pamper her. "The delivery was very hard, but after the delivery was a time of celebration and relaxation for the mother." In the US, she experienced disappointment when she came home from the hospital with her seventh baby and had no family there to greet her. "Here the delivery is very easy, but then you go home to just your husband and your other children, and that is the saddest part." Separated from her village of support, Hamida experiences child rearing alone for the first time. This leaves her with acute feelings of isolation and loss.

Power structures exist in all families, between partners, parents and their children, and within multigenerational households. The informal roles taken on by each family member are often disrupted during resettlement and can cause tension in familial relationships.

School-aged children learn English more easily and become acculturated faster than their parents or older siblings. This may lead to children serving as informal interpreters for their family members in a variety of settings. Not only does this upset the power difference that typically exists between parents and their children but it also gives children access to sensitive information from which parents may have preferred to shield their children. Minor children should never be used as interpreters in health care settings, and this practice is prohibited by law.[3]

Within multigenerational immigrant families, the new role of breadwinner may place adult children in positions of power over their parents, upending the traditional family dynamics from their country of origin. Older immigrants, those with low literacy, and those without technological skills have the most difficulties acculturating.[20] These individuals are also the least likely to engage with their health care providers independently, as they often rely on younger relatives with more English proficiency to act as informal health care navigators on their behalf.[21] Feelings of isolation can become prominent in older immigrants, who may be home alone while their children are at work and their grandchildren are at school.

Feelings of isolation are also prominent in female immigrants. In their countries of origin, women had access to wide social networks through family, tribes, and communities, even if they did not hold jobs outside of the home. In the US these relations are interrupted by distance, unfamiliar transportation systems, and the addition of new roles, including work outside of the home. Women may feel this changing dynamic most acutely after the birth of a child, as in the case of Hamida. A potential source of support for mothers and their newborns is a family member visiting from their country of origin with a B-2 tourist visa. Health care providers may be asked to provide a letter of support inviting the family member to visit in order to help care for the patient and her newborn; however, this is not a requirement and is not used by the US Department of State in determining whether to issue the visa.[22]

IMPACTS OF IMMIGRATION POLICY

> *Zabi is a refugee from Syria who arrived as a teenager with his siblings and mother 5 years ago. Zabi financially supports himself and his mother, as his mother is disabled and his older siblings have moved out of the home. Despite his full-time job, the family relies on rental assistance and the SNAP in order to afford housing, food, and bills. During a medical appointment, Zabi tells the RN care coordinator that he plans to call social services to discontinue his SNAP and housing assistance; he fears that accepting these benefits will render him ineligible for citizenship. Fortunately, the care coordinator was able to reassure Zabi that refugees are exempt from the Inadmissibility on Public Charge Grounds Rule,[23] and he did not cancel his benefits.*

Rapid and sweeping changes in immigration policy under the Trump administration have direct and indirect impacts on the health of immigrants. The 2017 announcement to rescind the Deferred Action for Childhood Arrivals (DACA) Program plunged hundreds of thousands of affected residents into uncertainty.[24] In the wake of the 2017 Executive Order 13769 "Protecting the Nation From Foreign Terrorist Entry Into the United States," also known as the "Muslim ban" or the "travel ban," Muslim immigrants reported feeling unwelcome, and this period has coincided with an increase in hate crimes.[25] Despite record numbers of refugees and internally displaced people the world over,[26] the US refugee resettlement ceiling for fiscal year 2020 is at its lowest in the 40 year history of the program, at 18,000.[27] The drastic decrease in the refugee resettlement ceiling has resulted in widespread resettlement agency closures, impairing the capacity to expand the resettlement program in the future.[28] Increases in Immigration and Customs Enforcement apprehensions and detentions, -including near schools and medical facilities, have sewn fear in immigrant communities, resulting in decreased utilization of health care and public services.[29]

The Inadmissibility on Public Charge Grounds Rule, also known as the "Public Charge Rule," deters immigrants from seeking assistance for which they may be eligible. At the US-Mexico border, changing demographics of immigrants and dramatic shifts in enforcement policies have led to a humanitarian crisis. Although most of the immigrants crossing the border have historically been single men seeking employment, most of the immigrants apprehended at the border in recent years have been families or unaccompanied children seeking asylum.[13] The "zero tolerance" policy of the Trump administration ensures prosecution for all persons crossing the US-Mexico border illegally. Consequently, immigrant children, who cannot legally be detained in federal criminal detention facilities, are separated from their families.[30] Crowded detention facilities and family separations add to the trauma that led asylum seekers to flee their home countries and to the trauma many experience en route to the US. Crowding at these facilities also raises concerns for the potential for infectious disease outbreaks in a vulnerable population.

LGBTQ ISSUES

> *Alejandra is a 38-year-old transgender female asylum-seeker from Honduras. She fled her home country due to multiple attempts on her life due to her gender identity. On crossing the US-Mexico border, she was apprehended by Immigration and Customs Enforcement and placed in a detention facility with male detainees. She was sexually assaulted on more than one occasion during her detainment and was placed in solitary confinement "for her protection." Medical evaluation conducted during her detention revealed that she is human immunodeficiency virus positive. During her first visit with her primary care physician, Alejandra is referred to an endocrinologist, infectious disease specialist, social worker, and psychologist.*

In order to be granted asylum based on sexual orientation or gender identity, an asylum-seeker must be able to prove to the Board of Immigration Appeals that they were being persecuted due to their sexual orientation or gender identity and that there is a systemic, pervasive, or organized pattern of persecuting such individuals in their country of origin.[31] The burden of proof can be particularly daunting when one considers that most asylum seekers do not have access to legal representation.[32] LGBTQ asylum seekers may face trauma during detainment in the US, including assault by other detainees and the psychological trauma of solitary confinement.

Although gender identity or sexual orientation can form the basis for the designation of refugee status, this may not be disclosed to resettlement agencies. It is also very likely that an LBGTQ refugee or asylee was granted this status for reasons other than gender identity or sexual orientation. LGBTQ refugees and asylees may be particularly isolated owing to having been persecuted by their own family or community and due to fears of discrimination in the US. It is important for health care providers to actively support LGBTQ individuals by providing affirming care and clearly communicating that theirs is a safe space.[33] Transgender immigrants are a particularly vulnerable group due to high rates of discrimination, mental illness, chronic disease, and limited access to affirming health care.[34–37]

economic fallout of the COVID-19 pandemic unfolds, immigrants will likely become more vulnerable to vilification. Indeed, Asian Americans have already been subjected to an increase in discrimination and harassment as a consequence of moral panic spurred by the pandemic.[47] Those of us who work closely with immigrants have the privilege of being able to advocate for this diverse, resilient population by

- Creating safe spaces[33]
- Redirecting attention to the underlying structural causes of inequality concealed by moral panic[42]
- Volunteering to provide medical asylum evaluations[48]
- Sharing the stories of immigrants[49]
- Partnering with a local legal services agency to form a medical-legal partnership[50]

SUMMARY

Immigrants to the US are a diverse group that has overcome significant hurdles in search of a better life. They enrich the US through economic contributions and unique perspectives. Immigrants find themselves navigating a new culture, a complicated health care system, unfamiliar social programs, and an ever-changing policy environment. They may be discouraged by unmet expectations of life in the US, changing family dynamics, and discrimination. Health care providers can assist and empower immigrants to navigate these challenges.

CLINICS CARE POINTS

- Assess the patient's and their family's understanding of their condition, health literacy, and expectations for treatment.
- Some immigrants are accustomed to a paternalistic style of care delivery and may be slow to engage in shared decision-making. Be sure to invite the patient to ask questions.
- Take the time at the initial clinic visit to explain how the clinic will communicate with the patient and to make sure the patient knows how to call the clinic and request an interpreter.
- Although the CDC provides guidance for a catch-up immunization schedule, refer to your local health department for state-specific vaccine requirements for school enrollment.
- Always offer professional interpretation, even if an English-speaking family member is present. Never use a minor child as an interpreter.
- Support LGBTQ individuals by providing affirming care and clearly communicating that yours is a safe space.

DISCLOSURE

The authors have nothing to disclose.

REFERENCES

1. Kleinman A. The illness narratives: suffering, healing, and the human condition. New York: Basic Books; 1998.
2. What is Health Literacy? Centers for Disease Control and Prevention. Available at: https://www.cdc.gov/healthliteracy/learn/index.html. Accessed June 1, 2020.

3. Jacobs B, Ryan AM, Henrichs KS, et al. Medical Interpreters in Outpatient Practice. Ann Fam Med 2018;16(1):70–6.

4. About the Voluntary Agencies Matching Grant Program. Office of Refugee Resettlement. Available at: https://www.acf.hhs.gov/orr/programs/matching-grants/about. Accessed June 1, 2020.

5. From Struggle to resilience: the economic Impact of Refugees in America. New American Economy; 2017. Available at: https://www.newamericaneconomy.org/wp-content/uploads/2017/06/NAE_Refugees_V5.pdf.

6. Blau FD, Mackie C, editors. The economic and fiscal consequences of immigration. Washington, DC: The National Academies Press; 2017.

7. Aurand A, Cooper A, Emmanuel D, et al. Out of reach 2019. Washington, DC: National Low Income Housing Coalition; 2019.

8. Housing Choice Vouchers Fact Sheet. U.S. Department of Housing and Urban Development. Available at: https://www.hud.gov/program_offices/public_indian_housing/programs/hcv/about/fact_sheet. Accessed June 1, 2020.

9. Immigrant Rights. National Housing Law Project. Available at: https://www.nhlp.org/initiatives/immigrant-rights/. Accessed June 1, 2020.

10. Turner MA, Santos R, Levy DK, et al. Housing discrimination against racial and ethnic minorities 2012. Washington, DC: US Department of Housing and Urban Development; 2013.

11. Auspurg K, Schneck A, Hinz T. Closed doors everywhere? A meta-analysis of field experiments on ethnic discrimination in rental housing markets. J Ethn Migr Stud 2019;45(1):95–114.

12. Refugee Statistics. United Nations High Commissioner for Refugees. Available at: https://www.unrefugees.org/refugee-facts/statistics/. Accessed June 1, 2020.

13. Capps R, Meissner D, Soto AGR, et al. From control to crisis: changing trends and policies reshaping U.S.-Mexico border enforcement. Washington, DC: Migration Policy Institute; 2019.

14. Vaccination Technical Instructions for Civil Surgeons. 2017. Available at: https://www.cdc.gov/immigrantrefugeehealth/exams/ti/civil/vaccination-civil-technical-instructions.html. Accessed June 1, 2020.

15. Information for Limited English Proficient (LEP) Parents and Guardians and for Schools and School Districts that Communicate with Them. U.S. Department of Justice and U.S. Department of Education. 2015. Available at: https://www2.ed.gov/about/offices/list/ocr/docs/dcl-factsheet-lep-parents-201501.pdf. Accessed June 1, 2020.

16. School and day care minimum immunization requirements. Virginia Department of Health. Available at: https://www.vdh.virginia.gov/immunization/requirements/. Accessed July 31, 2020.

17. The future of refugee Welcome in the United States. Washington, DC: International Rescue Committee; 2017. Available at: https://www.rescue.org/sites/default/files/document/1872/policybriefthefutureofrefugeewelcome.pdf.

18. Roxas K. Tales from the front lines: Teachers' responses to Somali Bantu refugee students. Urban Educ 2011;46(3):513–48.

19. Solberg MA, Peters RM. Adverse childhood experiences in non-westernized nations: Implications for immigrant and refugee health. J Immigr Minor Health 2020; 22:145–55.

20. Banulescu-Bogdan N. Beyond work: reducing social isolation for refugee women and other marginalized newcomers. Washington, DC: Migration Policy Institute; 2020.

37. Belranet S, Raisal T, Keatley A, et al. Global health burden and needs of transgender populations: a review. Lancet 2016;388(10042):412–36.

38. COVID-19 in racial and ethnic minority groups. Centers for Disease Control and Prevention. 2020. Available at: https://www.cdc.gov/coronavirus/2019-ncov/need-extra-precautions/racial-ethnic-minorities.html. Accessed June 4, 2020.

39. Travelers' Health. Centers for Disease Control and Prevention. Available at: https://wwwnc.cdc.gov/travel. Accessed June 5, 2020.

40. I am a lawful permanent resident of 5 years. US Citizenship and Immigration Services. Available at: https://www.uscis.gov/citizenship/learn-about-citizenship/citizenship-and-naturalization/i-am-a-lawful-permanent-resident-of-5-years. Accessed July 31, 2020.

41. N-648, medical certification for disability exceptions. U.S. Citizenship and Immigration Services. Available at: https://www.uscis.gov/n-648. Accessed June 1, 2020.

42. Evetsman MH, Bird JDP. Moral injury and social justice: A guide for analyzing social problems. Soc Work 2017;62(1):29–36.

43. Remarks by President Trump on the illegal immigration crisis and border security. The White House. Available at: https://www.whitehouse.gov/briefings-statements/remarks-president-trump-illegal-immigration-crisis-border-security/. Accessed June 1, 2020.

44. Nielsen KM. Policy guidance for implementation of the migrant protection protocols. Washington, DC: US Department of Homeland Security; 2019.

45. Transactional Records Access Clearinghouse. Available at: https://trac.syr.edu/phptools/immigration/mpp/. Accessed July 31, 2020.

46. Munro A. Asylum-seekers stranded in Mexico face homelessness, kidnapping, and sexual violence. ACLU. Available at: ... immigrants-rights ... Accessed July 31, 2020.

47. ... in the LGBTQ+ pandemic ... A call for research, practice, and policy responses. Psychol Trauma 2020;12:H1–H3.

Models of Health Care: Interprofessional Approaches to Serving Immigrant Populations

Catherine E. Elmore, PhD(c), MSN, RN, CNL[a],*,
Rebekah Compton, DNP, RN, FNP-C[b], Erica Uhlmann, MPH[c]

KEYWORDS

- Delivery of health care • Immigrants • Refugees • Asylum seekers • North America

KEY POINTS

- Developing a model of care to serve immigration populations requires an understanding of population- and individual-level factors that impact health care delivery.
- An ideal model of care consists of a team of interprofessional clinicians working together with community partners; team growth over time should be supported to meet emerging needs.
- Community and population assessments are important to identify resources and challenges, and models of care should aim to address local needs.
- Clinical operations should include processes for obtaining patient consent to communicate among community partners, scheduling extended appointments, and ensuring language access for appointment scheduling.
- Providing cultural sensitivity training and ongoing work to build trust and sustain relationships with the community are essential parts of an ideal care model.

INTRODUCTION

Developing an integrated model of health care for refugees, asylees, and immigrants, and special immigrant visa holders (hereinafter collectively referred to as "immigrants") requires a multifaceted approach because of unique and complex health care needs. There are population- and individual-level factors to care that need to be addressed. Although this may seem overwhelming because of common challenges related to limited clinical staffing and financial constraints, having a structured

[a] School of Nursing, University of Virginia, PO Box 800729, Charlottesville, VA 22908, USA;
[b] Department of Family Medicine, University of Virginia, PO Box 800729, Charlottesville, VA 22908, USA; [c] International Rescue Committee, 609 East Market Street, Suite 104, Charlottesville, VA 22902, USA
* Corresponding author.
E-mail address: ceh9s@virginia.edu

Prim Care Clin Office Pract 48 (2021) 163–177
https://doi.org/10.1016/j.pop.2020.10.003
0095-4543/21/© 2020 Elsevier Inc. All rights reserved.
primarycare.theclinics.com

approach for providing adequate resources to address the various needs is beneficial to the care team and the patients. The purpose of this article is to

1. Illuminate population- and individual-level factors important to caring for immigrant populations
2. Provide guidance on creating a model of care that addresses these factors
3. Describe established clinics that exemplify strong models of care

IMPORTANT FACTORS WHEN CARING FOR IMMIGRANT POPULATIONS

It is helpful to understand the range of factors, representing barriers and needs, the immigrant population currently faces when accessing health care services in countries of resettlement. Some of the factors listed here are not unique to immigrants, but all present genuine challenges and additional burdens that should be considered.

- Navigating new health care systems: Identifying who will see them, how to contact clinics and set up appointments can seem overwhelming, especially when they may need to access care after hours to avoid losing their employment or obtaining child care.
- Trust: There may also be a sense of mistrust among families as they enter this new and unknown system of health care.[1]
- Cultural considerations: Immigrants come from a variety of backgrounds and cultures with various attitudes, beliefs, and practices regarding health care.[2] There may be differences with their customary approach to health care compared with Western medicine.
- Unrealistic expectations and understanding of Western medicine[3]: For some, there is a belief that the Western doctors are going to cure their family members of serious health conditions, some of which are genetic and/or incurable. Or there may be unrealistic expectations about cost of care; as an example, a couple may assume effective fertility treatments are easy to access in the United States and do not realize Medicaid does not cover the cost of treatments.
- Countries of origin may be resource poor: Many immigrants have health conditions (especially chronic conditions) that were poorly controlled, managed, and treated in their home country, in the country where they were displaced before moving to the United States, or in refugee camps.
- Sharing medical records/ensuring continuity of care: Immigrants of all kinds may not have copies of past medical records on establishment of care, which means that piecing together past medical, surgical, and immunization history may be difficult or frustrating. By the same token, these individuals may leave your practice at some point in the future, so we recommend setting up a system to enable them to obtain records and clearly communicate their health care needs with their next health care providers.
- Language access: Immigrants with limited English proficiency benefit when professional medical interpreters are used in health care settings.[4] In the United States, Title VI of the Civil Rights Act mandates the provision of language access to organizations that accept federal funding; in the case of health care, this applies to Medicaid and Medicare.[5] Beyond the legal obligation, the moral obligation to provide linguistically appropriate care reaps vast benefits. The use of trained interpreters results in fewer communication errors and enhances the patient care delivery and experience (discussed Joseph S. Tan and Claudia W. Allen's article, "Cultural Considerations in Caring for Refugees and Immigrants," elsewhere in this issue).[6,7]

- Insurance and medical expenses: The inability to qualify for or afford health insurance coverage, coverage gaps, and costs related to copays and coinsurance are common barriers for immigrants.[8] It may also impact the quality of health care services received. Even for refugees who are eligible for Medicaid, delays in approval can also be detrimental to urgent care needs.[9]
- Low health literacy skills: Some immigrants have a poorer understanding of their medical condition, impaired medication compliance, and poor follow through with instructions for treatments and medical procedures. For example, for those who had never been exposed to cancer screening in their country of origin, we have found that a clear, thoughtful, and comprehensive instructional video in Nepali (one of our clinic's most common languages) to be most effective with improving adherence to colonoscopy preparation procedures and screening outcomes. Use of the video resulted in a decrease in canceled procedures and a reduction in lost clinic income.
- Logistical issues: Transportation is a universal barrier, because those who rely on public transportation to attend appointments are limited by routes and hours of operation.[8] Child care, clinic hours of service outside of patient working hours, long wait times for appointments, and the inability to be seen as a walk-in patient are also common logistical barriers. Additionally, many immigrants face a lack of autonomy at work making it difficult to get time off for appointments.
- Obtaining medications: Lack of insurance, or a change in coverage or formularies, can make it difficult to access or afford medications. This, along with language barriers and lack of interpreter services at pharmacies, can result in patients not obtaining medications or understanding medication instructions, further contributing to poorly managed care and less than optimal outcomes.

GUIDANCE ON CREATING A MODEL CLINIC FOR IMMIGRANT POPULATIONS

This section provides guidance on creating models of care to address the well-documented needs to health care access faced by immigrants.[10] Community assessments can further identify and clarify barriers that are specific to a particular community or population.

Start Small and Let Local Needs Drive Growth

We recommend a model of care that consists of an interprofessional team working together with community partners.[11] As with any process, it is important to start small and add on resources as your clinical model becomes more stable and further needs and community partners are identified. For example, at the University of Virginia, the initial care model started with two physicians, a nurse practitioner, and a social worker.[11] Over a span of nearly 10 years, and with multiple iterations, additional clinicians, including behavioral health specialists, psychiatrists, specialty physicians, resident physicians, a registered nurse care coordinator (RNCC), a designated social worker, and a clinical pharmacist were added to make up the now-existing team structure. **Fig. 1** depicts this model of care showing interaction between interprofessional clinical team members and community organizations as they partner to support immigrant patients.

Importance of Community Assessment and Collaboration

When identifying how and where to start, it is extremely useful to determine the population to be served and to conduct a community health needs assessment.[12] The Centers for Disease Control and Prevention recommends several frameworks for

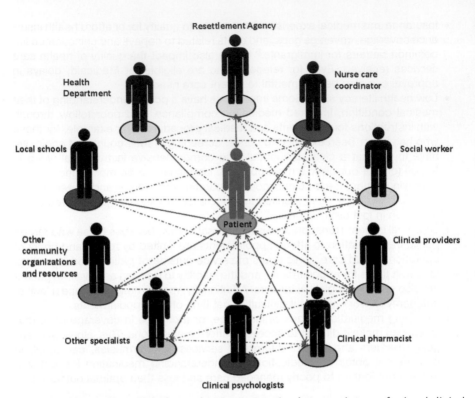

Fig. 1. Depiction of a model of care showing interaction between interprofessional clinical team members and community organizations as they partner to support immigrant patients. (*Courtesy of* K. O. Tanabe, MPH, Charlottesville, VA.)

conducting a community health needs assessment, and others have provided helpful guiding principles.[13,14] Although the community health needs assessment may cast a larger net and identify multiple care gaps among various community groups, the information gathered in an assessment helps identify organizations and individuals from within the community to include as the model of care is developed. Information is gathered via simple surveys or calls to local health departments, departments of social services, free clinics, resettlement agencies, public schools, and legal aid centers. Other sources of information can include organizations serving low-income members in the community, such as food banks and donation centers, because they have a sense of who is needing services.

Understanding your community resources, such as transportation, volunteer organizations, free clinics, and other health care networks, is vital. Other members from the community to include are public school staff: teachers, school nurses, and English as a second language coordinators. Establishing these connections across the community is imperative to share and address challenges and resources community partners have identified.

As the internal team is building, additional community connections must be made and maintained. An example of this includes hosting quarterly meetings with community stakeholders and inviting others, on an as-needed basis, to discuss population needs and specific patient needs.[11,15] Consider using these meetings to educate the team on trends in new arrivals to the community, including strengths and challenges that a certain group may face. This allows the team to be prepared to assist in identifying solutions.

Essential Personnel to Include in a Model Clinic

Here, we consider essential components of the team care model, but communities differ in their presentation and as such, so do the teams created to meet those needs.

Primary point of contact

A day-to-day primary point of contact at the clinic should be identified to enhance the communication between the clinic and various collaborative partners, including the patients themselves. Ideally, this primary point of contact is a capable clinician who has the ability to assess and triage patient health needs, assist with clinical decision making, and coordinate care within the health system and with community partners.

When the University of Virginia Family Medicine implemented an RNCC as the primary point of contact, this clinician was able to streamline communication, reduce ad hoc contacts to multiple providers, and improve responsiveness to time-sensitive problems, thereby saving time and cost. The RNCC expedites the process of triaging patient needs, before and in the initial months after arrival. This is done by consulting with resettlement agency medical case managers and by examining overseas medical records. Time frame for initial appointments can be adjusted, referrals can be made for urgent needs, and unnecessary visits to the emergency department can be reduced when needs are triaged appropriately.[16] These objectives are more difficult to achieve by a nonclinician staff member in the role. However, if an RN or another clinician is not a resource that is available, a medical assistant or access/registration staff can also assist in this triage process in collaboration with a designated clinician who would be responsible for clinical decision making.

In addition, the primary point of contact can improve ongoing communication related to special medical cases and subsequent follow-up needs by communicating with the resettlement agency about referrals and follow-up appointments. This helps to ensure timely scheduling of follow-up, transportation, and clinic wayfinding, thereby reducing no-shows and improving continuity of care. The primary point of contact serves as an advocate, educator, and resource to reduce delays in care to help improve the patients' ability to successfully navigate the health care system.

Language interpreters

Clinics and health systems who care for diverse populations must provide access to interpretation for all languages spoken by their patient population. When language concordant providers are not available, professionally trained language interpreters (either in-person or by telephone or video) become essential team members in the model clinic. Interpreters play an important role in helping health care workers identify and interpret cultural nuances, and identify subtle differences in understanding between patients and families and their health care providers.[17] Ideally, interpreters should not be family members, particularly because of sensitive medical information being shared. Children should never be asked to interpret for family members, because this is ethically problematic and places an undue burden on them.[6] The authors are aware that language discordance is a common challenge that the clinical team will be confronted with and find that setting expectations and investing in the necessary resources from the beginning prevents this from being an ongoing issue.

diet in a new country. For example, Bhutanese refugees who lived on lentils, rice, and dried fish rations in camps before resettlement may find it difficult to consider experimenting with new-to-them vegetables or restraining their children's intake of sugar-laden foods. Although we caution against categorical generalizations about cultural groups,[22] such culture-specific knowledge can lead to more direct education to help prevent illnesses that may result from these decisions.

Throughout the process, supporting the educational needs of all clinician learners is important. These learners are considered part of the model of care and provide important contributions in the way of gathering information and data, and writing reports describing information that is already available or is needed as it relates to any given issue. Engaging our learners as part of the team increases comfort level with knowledge of immigrant health, overall enjoyment caring for these patients, and interest in caring for immigrant populations in their future work.[23]

Building trust

Building trust and earning respect of the patient and even larger community is of utmost importance as the clinic establishes a model of care to support the various patient populations.[24] Unfortunately, mistrust has been already established for many of these individuals as they have had to navigate complex health care systems or have endured a lack of support from health care systems or other public service systems. Providing care team education on the different cultures and population needs assists in bridging this gap. Identifying ways to support cultural preferences, as long as safety is not compromised, is encouraged. Where this is a challenge is when cultural norms for one society clash with legal systems in another, such as with young teenage girls marrying at the age of 14 and 15. Although this may be a common or at least possible practice in some countries, it is not legal in the United States. Similarly, female circumcision is permitted in some countries and is not in the United States. In both these situations cultural sensitivity is necessary while educating the parties involved to help them understand potential consequences if acted on while living in the United States.

Training is needed bidirectionally so that health care workers receive the necessary training as it pertains to patients' cultural needs, but for patients to also receive an orientation or educational session on understanding and navigating the Western culture. This information should also include guidance on accessing the health care system.

Considerations for Asylum Claimants and Undocumented Immigrants

Provision of health care for asylum claimants and undocumented immigrants requires overcoming unique barriers, including legal barriers. Because these individuals may delay seeking care because of fear of legal repercussions,[25] model clinics should consider implementing policies that encourage attendance and do not discourage attendance by these individuals and families. Policies that encourage attendance include the provision of legal services in the health care setting (as is the case with medical-legal partnerships). In addition to the need for access to usual care, asylum claimants in Canada and the United States are required to undergo health and legal assessments as they apply for refugee status. In the United States, clinics can staff Civil Surgeons who are authorized by US Citizenship and Immigration Services to conduct medical examinations that contribute to asylum seekers' applications for refugee status. Policies that do not discourage attendance include not requiring patients to disclose their legal status and not recording status in the medical record if known to the provider.

Clinics may consider opening up a dialogue and partnering with local employers of undocumented migrant farm workers to ensure that these workers know about available services, but also to assess population-level needs, such as education and risk mitigation around environmental toxins (e.g. pesticides) that workers may be exposed to in their work environment.

Clinicians should be aware of variations in local, state, and national policies related to accessing social system benefits for these individuals.[25] For example, in the United States there may be limited coverage by emergency Medicaid, but access to chronic treatment, such as dialysis for end-stage renal disease, varies by state.[25] Barriers to coverage may be fewer for children in some states.[25] Other challenges for clinicians and patients include lack of access to historical medical records, and no way to obtain past medical and vaccination history.[26] Clinicians should be aware that some immigrants speak local dialects, creating additional challenges in overcoming language barriers.[26]

EXAMPLES OF ESTABLISHED CLINICS THAT EXEMPLIFY STRONG MODELS OF CARE
Fully Established Integrated Models

An integrated model is beneficial not only because patients have an established medical home, but they also have access to a comprehensive and diverse range of health care services and a support team. We identified several examples of models of care for immigrant populations throughout the United States. **Table 1** summarizes key features of these six models. Note that the characteristics are shown only to the extent that we could find evidence of them in the published literature. These clinics may have features that are not captured on this table.

Medical-Legal Partnerships

Medical-legal partnerships are a model of care that connects health care teams with lawyers and paralegals to identify, address, and prevent health-harming legal needs for individuals and populations.[27] Medical-legal partnerships are ideal models for addressing the unique needs of asylum seekers and undocumented immigrants.

Measuring Outcomes

There are many positive outcomes from implementing these models of care, which are significant and worth mentioning. Forsyth County, North Carolina, experienced a decline in emergency room visits; better planning for medical care prearrival; and improved communication, access to community resources, and provider and family education.[28] Philadelphia's Collaborative successfully connected refugee patients to a patient-centered medical home where management of chronic diseases improved and there was overall improved access to preventive care services, including a decrease in the average wait time for initial health screening appointments.[15] Hasbro Children's Hospital's Clinic experienced increased screening rates for tuberculosis, human immunodeficiency virus, hepatitis B, and elevated blood lead, and increased the rate of latent tuberculosis treatment among children.[29]

CONSIDERATIONS FOR VULNERABLE POPULATIONS IN A CHANGING HEALTH CARE ENVIRONMENT

The most recent coronavirus pandemic events have underscored the need for comprehensive health care teams, especially for vulnerable populations. With the expansion of telehealth as a way to bridge health care needs, this evolution further identified the gaps in health care to ensure those without technology

Table 1
(continued)

Reference Describing Clinic:	Bosson et al,[30] 2017	Divito et al,[15] 2016, Wendel,[31] 2013	Elmore et al,[11] 2019	Michael et al,[28] 2019	Reavy et al,[32] 2012	Temu et al,[29] 2012
Preappointment orientation to health care system		X				
Treats IDs and NCDs		X	X			X
Adult focus			X			
Pediatric and adolescent focus			X			X
Registry of patients			X	X		
Ongoing community needs assessment						X

Abbreviations: C.A.R.E., culturally appropriate resources and education; HD, health department; ID, infectious disease; NCD, noncommunicable disease; RA, resettlement agency; X, key feature present in model.

support, Internet access, or language support could continue to access the same level of care as those fortunate to have these resources. Having the ability to identify the population through panel management provides the opportunity for a clinical team to arrange specific outreach for those who are more vulnerable, may not have the previously mentioned resources, and consider alternative ways to manage their care. However, even if the population can be identified, further measures are needed at a much higher health care system level to support those individuals who are at highest risk of being lost to care. As our government, societies, and world implement changes to meet the new demands of health care, we need to continue to advocate for the most vulnerable people who are unable to speak up for themselves.

SUMMARY

This article has illuminated population- and individual-level factors important to caring for immigrant populations, provided guidance on creating a model of care that addresses these factors, and described established clinics that exemplify strong models of care. The authors note a lack of shared knowledge regarding various models of care that may and do exist in North America. Through personal conversations and presentations at conferences, we know that others have developed different models to address the populations in their community. Unfortunately, little has been published on those models and we suspect there are many more of which we are unaware. We hope that through sharing our experience and findings, other systems will be encouraged to do the same so that the models of care being delivered to address the health care needs of refugees, asylees, and immigrants can be improved and enhanced. Finally, the models that we have depicted here are models of care that would be appropriate for all vulnerable populations and can be adapted to fit identified care needs.

CLINICS CARE POINTS

- Identify a capable clinician within the clinic who can be a primary point of contact to enhance day-to-day communication between community partners, including the patients themselves.

- Develop partnerships among the community, within and outside of your clinic's organization, by creating opportunities for regular meetings and discussion about population and patient needs.

- Promote cultural sensitivity among team members to allow for enhanced understanding of cultural nuances and differences that may impact health care needs and knowledge.

- Establish trusting relationships to reduce barriers among providers, clinical care teams, and patients and thereby promote communication and support of ongoing care needs.

- Use professionally trained medical interpreters for all clinic encounters to ensure accurate, and appropriate, communication between patient and provider.

DISCLOSURE

The authors have nothing to disclose.

REFERENCES

1. Mangrio E, Sjögren Forss K. Refugees' experiences of healthcare in the host country: a scoping review. BMC Health Serv Res 2017;17(1):814.
2. Fabio M, Parker LD, Siddharth MB. Building on resiliencies of refugee families. Pediatr Clin North Am 2019;66(3):655–67.
3. Robertshaw L, Dhesi S, Jones LL. Challenges and facilitators for health professionals providing primary healthcare for refugees and asylum seekers in high-income countries: a systematic review and thematic synthesis of qualitative research. BMJ Open 2017;7(8):e015981.
4. Karliner LS, Jacobs EA, Chen AH, et al. Do professional interpreters improve clinical care for patients with limited English proficiency? A systematic review of the literature. Health Serv Res 2007;42(2):727–54.
5. Title VI Of The Civil Rights Act Of 1964 42 U.S.C. § 2000d Et Seq. Available at: https://www.justice.gov/crt/fcs/TitleVI-Overview. Accessed June 8, 2020.
6. Juckett G, Unger K. Appropriate use of medical interpreters. Am Fam Physician 2014;90(7):476–80.
7. Rasi, S. 2020. Impact of Language Barriers on Access to Healthcare Services by Immigrant Patients: A systematic review. Asia Pacific Journal of Health Management. 15, 1 (Mar. 2020), 35-48. https://doi.org/10.24083/apjhm.v15i1.271.
8. Morris MD, Popper ST, Rodwell TC, et al. Healthcare barriers of refugees post-resettlement. J Community Health 2009;34(6):529–38.
9. Morillo JR. Connecting newly arrived refugees to health care in North Carolina. N C Med J 2019;80(2):89–93.
10. Batista R, Pottie K, Bouchard L, et al. Primary health care models addressing health equity for immigrants: a systematic scoping review. J Immigr Minor Health 2018;20(1):214–30.
11. Elmore CE, Tingen JM, Fredgren K, et al. Using an interprofessional team to provide refugee healthcare in an academic medical centre. Fam Med Commun Hlth 2019;7(3):e000091.
12. CDC. Assessment and plans - community health assessment. Available at: https://www.cdc.gov/publichealthgateway/cha/plan.html. Accessed June 9, 2020.
13. CDC. Assessment & planning models, frameworks & tools. Public Health Professionals Gateway. 2015. Available at: https://www.cdc.gov/publichealthgateway/cha/assessment.html. Accessed June 9, 2020.
14. Rosenbaum S. Principles to consider for the implementation of a community health needs assessment process. Washington, DC: George Washington University; 2013.
15. Divito B, Payton C, Shanfeld G, et al. A collaborative approach to promoting continuing care for refugees: Philadelphia's strategies and lessons learned. Harv Health Policy Rev 2016;9:1–12.
16. Guess MA, Tanabe KO, Nelson AE, et al. Emergency department and primary care use by refugees compared to non-refugee controls. J Immigr Minor Health 2019;21:793–800.
17. Hsieh E, Kramer EM. Medical interpreters as tools: dangers and challenges in the utilitarian approach to interpreters' roles and functions. Patient Educ Couns 2012; 89(1):158–62.
18. Shommu NS, Ahmed S, Rumana N, et al. What is the scope of improving immigrant and ethnic minority healthcare using community navigators: a systematic scoping review. Int J Equity Health 2016;15:6.

19. Hartzler AL, Tuzzio L, Hsu C, et al. Roles and functions of community health workers in primary care. Ann Fam Med 2018;16(3):240–5.
20. Thompson RH, Snyder AE, Burt DR, et al. Risk screening for cardiovascular disease and diabetes in Latino migrant farmworkers: a role for the community health worker. J Community Health 2015;40(1):131–7.
21. Eckstein B. Primary care for refugees. Am Fam Physician 2011;83(4):429–36.
22. Jongen C, McCalman J, Bainbridge R. Health workforce cultural competency interventions: a systematic scoping review. BMC Health Serv Res 2018;18(1):232.
23. Alpern JD, Davey CS, Song J. Perceived barriers to success for resident physicians interested in immigrant and refugee health. BMC Med Educ 2016;16:178.
24. Brandenberger J, Tylleskär T, Sontag K, et al. A systematic literature review of reported challenges in health care delivery to migrants and refugees in high-income countries: the 3C model. BMC Public Health 2019;19(1):755.
25. Fernández A, Rodriguez RA. Undocumented immigrants and access to health care. JAMA Intern Med 2017;177(4):536–7.
26. Lopez-Murray E. Health of asylum-seeking immigrants: providing medical care from a volunteer's perspective. JAAPA 2019;32(8):13–4.
27. Williamson A, Trott J, Regenstein M. Health-center based medical-legal partnerships: where they are, how they work, and how they are funded. George Washington University: Washington DC, National Center for Medical-Legal Partnership; 2018.
28. Michael L, Brady AK, Russell G, et al. Connecting refugees to medical homes through multi-sector collaboration. J Immigr Minor Health 2019;21(1):198–203.
29. Temu TM, Ratanaprasatporn L, Ratanaprasatporn L, et al. The patient-centered medical home for refugee children in Rhode Island. Int J Popul Res 2012; 2012:1–6.
30. Bosson R, Carrico RM, Raghuram A, et al. Refugee-centered medical home: a new approach to care at the University of Louisville Global Health Center. RGH 2017;1(1). https://doi.org/10.18297/rgh/vol1/iss1/3/.
31. Wendel G. Philadelphia Refugee Health Collaborative. Social Innovations Journal 2013;13. Available at: https://socialinnovationsjournal.org/76-featured-social-innovations/811-philadelphia-refugee-health-collaborative. Accessed April 15, 2020.
32. Reavy K, Hobbs J, Hereford M, et al. A new clinic model for refugee health care: adaptation of cultural safety. Rural Remote Health 2012;12:1826.

Moving?

Make sure your subscription moves with you!

To notify us of your new address, find your **Clinics Account Number** (located on your mailing label above your name), and contact customer service at:

Email: journalscustomerservice-usa@elsevier.com

800-654-2452 (subscribers in the U.S. & Canada)
314-447-8871 (subscribers outside of the U.S. & Canada)

Fax number: 314-447-8029

**Elsevier Health Sciences Division
Subscription Customer Service
3251 Riverport Lane
Maryland Heights, MO 63043**

*To ensure uninterrupted delivery of your subscription,
please notify us at least 4 weeks in advance of move.